The Myth of Osteoporosis

Gillian Sanson

No part of this book is intended to substitute for medical advice, diagnosis, or treatment. Every individual is unique, and no book can possibly address each person's special situation. Do not make changes in your medications or lifestyle without consulting your health care provider. The information contained in this book is intended to stimulate discussion with your health care providers, and not to replace their advice.

Printed on acid-free paper by Cushing-Malloy, Inc. Printed in U.S.A.

2nd Printing: August, 2004.

Cover Design: Ko Wicke, Black Dog Design.

For My Parents,
And For All the Members of My Wonderful Family

———————————

Table of Contents

Acknowledgements

The following people have generously offered invaluable information and resources. They have not been asked to endorse the contents of this book. My grateful thanks to: Dr. Susan Ott, Associate Professor of Medicine, University of Washington; Dr. Helen Roberts, Family Planning Research Manager and Senior Lecturer at Auckland University Medical School, New Zealand; Dr. Alan Tenenhouse, McGill University, Montreal; and Dr. Bruce Ettinger, Senior Investigator, Division of Research, Kaiser Permanente Medical Care Program, California. The family is grateful to Dr. Tim Cundy at the University of Auckland Medical School. His research into osteoporosis in young people is where our story really begins.

A special thanks to Dr. Arminée Kazanjian and her team at the British Columbia Office of Health Technology Assessment, whose pioneering review of the evidence for bone mineral testing has paved the way for a reconsideration of osteoporosis as it is currently defined, measured, and treated.

I am deeply grateful to Dr. Paul Dugliss for his commitment to making this book available to his patients and to all American women — without his insight and understanding of the issues around osteoporosis, it would not have happened. His re-creation of the structure and tone of this edition is masterful. And many thanks to Jordan Lubetkin, whose meticulous and thoughtful editing has fine-tuned and vastly improved the work.

Grateful thanks to Dr. Christiane Northrup for her generous endorsement, and for acknowledging the importance of educating women that a diagnosis of osteoporosis is not necessarily something to be feared.

Special thanks to dear friend Neil Hamill for his kindness, and his expertise in dealing with contractual agreements.

Finally, thanks to my wonderful parents and supportive extended family, who have been happy to have their stories told in the interests of helping others. I am especially grateful to Camille for allowing me to talk about her health so publicly, and to my sister Barbara for offering her personal experience as encouragement for others. My deepest gratitude to Stewart, who has supported me through every stage of this project.

Preface

When I first heard about Gill Sanson's book on osteoporosis, I was very excited. For years, I had been counseling women about issues of osteoporosis, wishing I had a book I could recommend that would present an accurate, evidenced-based view. Now I do.

With her well-researched work, Gill Sanson has done both the physician and the layperson a great service. She has provided clear insight into the myths of osteoporosis. These myths motivate both patient and physician into a lifetime of unnecessary testing and drug therapy — therapy that can in fact be life-threatening. Her well-documented explanation of these myths can spare women great anxiety. She takes the fear out of aging and restores women's sense of control over their bodies. She gives women good reasons for challenging the common way that osteoporosis is handled in the United States and in many other industrialized nations.

In this work, Gill Sanson explains many of the common myths of osteoporosis. She details how each has come to be and how women can avoid falling prey to them. These include:

- The myth that all women over the age of 50 are at risk for osteoporosis.

- The myth that osteoporosis is *the* cause of fractures in the elderly and that fractures in the elderly are deadly.

- The myth that the diagnosis of osteoporosis as a measure of low bone density is accurate, valid, and reliable.

- The myth that osteoporosis can be safely prevented and treated with drugs.

- The myth that taking drugs to increase one's bone mineral density necessarily decreases chances of a fracture.

- The myth that high calcium and dairy intake prevents osteoporosis.

Not only does this book correct many misconceptions, it provides positive steps women can take to create optimal bone health. It provides important information that women can use to take control of their future. It emphasizes the fact that bone health *can* be improved with exercise and lifestyle changes, and provides valuable dietary and nutritional information to help to keep bones strong. In creating a positive approach to the topic of osteoporosis, Gill Sanson has helped to eliminate a source of major concern for women who are going through or have been through menopause.

In many cultures, menopause is viewed as a natural and normal stage of life. Our Western view is different. Modern medicine has turned menopause into a syndrome that hallmarks the onset of increased health risk and loss. A major part of that syndrome is medicine's current approach to osteoporosis prevention. Unfortunately, that approach traps women into a complex system of ongoing technological assessment and treatment.

Nothing is so freeing as the truth. By exposing the myths of osteoporosis, Gill Sanson has set women free from worrying about bone loss. She has provided them with invaluable knowledge to maintain their health. And she does so in a way that reassures them about the wisdom of their own bodies. This is a book that I hope all the women in my practice will read.

Paul Dugliss, M.D.
Internist and Former Director,
Oakwood Healthcare System's
Complementary & Alternative Medicine Center

Section I: Major Myths

* I *
A Family Story

It was 1994, and I was relaxing in my New Zealand home, talking with guests, when my daughter rang from the Auckland Hospital fracture clinic. Camille, who was 16, had been having a follow-up visit for a wrist fracture sustained on the ski slopes a few weeks previously — her sixth fracture. It was the normal sort of teenage call: "I won't be home for a while," she said, "I am going into town to meet some friends." She added: "Oh, and by the way, the doctor who looked at my X-ray says that I have the bones of an 80-year-old."

I was speechless, devastated, and immediately stricken with guilt. I assumed Camille's condition was due to bad mothering, and I immediately started examining how I had raised her. Perhaps her condition arose because of an inadequate vegetarian diet lacking sufficient calcium. Or was it my diet during pregnancy that was at fault? I had always been conscientious about giving my children good food, but maybe I had made some critical mistake. My fears were irrational, of course, but I had many such questions and few answers. I was determined, however, to learn all I could about osteoporosis. That phone call became the impetus for this book.

In the meantime, Camille became justifiably frightened. She was young, alone, and had no context in which to gauge her diagnosis. Believing her fragile bones could not withstand any knocks or pressure, Camille immediately cut back on physical activity — conduct that was contrary to what she ought to have done, yet no such advice was given. (Years later, when I consider this event, I am appalled by the thoughtlessness of how she was told of her condition.)

Camille soon went for a bone densitometry scan, which confirmed that she had very low bone mineral density for her age. Extremely low bone density in young people is a concern because it means they haven't achieved the recognized, normal, healthy peak bone mass to take them through to adulthood and older age when bone density naturally declines and fracture risk increases. Initially, we were told that existing bone mass is like a bank account which can be drawn on. In Camille's case, according to current understanding, she was already in debt.

The family participated in a study at the endocrinology department at Auckland Hospital to determine a genetic risk factor. Measuring the bone densities of the entire extended family revealed that my three siblings, parents, husband, son, daughter, and I have varying degrees of low bone mineral density (BMD), culminating most seriously in my son and daughter. Six of us have osteoporosis, as defined by a BMD of −2.5 standard deviations (SD) below norm or less, and the rest of us have what is called osteopenia, or low bone density, a

BMD of −1 SD to −2.5 SDs. Males and females in the family are similarly afflicted, although none of us has fractured a bone since we were children — with the exception of my mother, who had a wrist fracture in her 60s. Growing up, my sister, brother, and I routinely broke wrists, the occasional digit, leg, or collarbone, and accepted that this was normal childhood wear and tear. In our small town of 14,000 inhabitants, we rather proudly held the record for the most X-rays at the local hospital. The fracturing eased off as we became adults, and when my children in turn started occasionally breaking their limbs, I stoically assumed the role of fracture-clinic mother, believing this was all a normal part of parenting.

Identifying idiopathic osteoporosis (osteoporosis of unknown origin) in our family raised many questions but provided no answers. Efforts to determine a cause were inconclusive. Blood DNA samples from individuals in the family and other similarly affected families were sent to Oxford, England, to screen for a common genetic factor. Researchers determined that there was a genetic link — though they were unsuccessful in isolating such a gene.[1]

For my children it was difficult to know what action to take. There wasn't any known treatment for very low bone density in a young person. All the tested, prescribed treatments were for postmenopausal women with low bone density. Hormonal treatments were inappropriate (like other healthy young women, my daughter's estrogen and progesterone levels were normal), and it wasn't clear that non-hormonal treatments would be effective in a person her age. I also remained unconvinced that the recommended drug (a bisphosphonate) would be safe, given the current lack of data on its use in young people.

Some family members had high levels of antibodies in their blood, which could indicate gluten intolerance or celiac disease. Celiac disease is known to be a "secondary" risk factor for osteoporosis, as it causes the villi (finger-like projections) in the wall of the small bowel to atrophy or disappear, thereby limiting the absorption of essential minerals. It is believed that maybe one in 130 people have this condition, often without realizing it — particularly those of Celtic origin, such as my family. The four of us in my immediate family embarked on a gluten-free diet — one of the recommended treatments for people who have celiac disease. After 18 months, our bone density remained unchanged.

I began to look deeper into possible causes of osteoporosis, ever conscious that the years when peak bone mass is established in a young person (up to about age 20) were almost over for my children. Camille's situation was identified as more serious than her brother's. His bone mass was low, though hers was significantly lower. Further, a young female can be at risk for additional bone loss during pregnancy and may lose bone mass more rapidly after menopause.

> *I didn't set out to write a provocative book on osteoporosis. I set out to find accurate information.*

Primarily, this book is the result of my search to uncover answers for the members of my family who have this diagnosis — relatives such as my oldest sister, now postmenopausal, who had experienced increased loss of bone density in her spine, yet found herself in the difficult position of having to make treatment decisions on the basis of little information.

When I began my research, I quickly learned that members of my family were not the only ones who were worried about their bone health. As a women's health educator, I conduct seminars and workshops in the community to help women manage the menopause transition and stay well in the years to follow. The subject of osteoporosis always surfaced in my classes, evoking feelings of anxiety and fear among many women who were convinced that they were candidates for osteoporosis by virtue of their age alone, once they passed through menopause. For most women, the question was not whether they were at risk for osteoporosis, but what to do about the impending condition. I would later discover that the widespread notion that all women are at risk for osteoporosis is a myth — though not the only one.

In these discussions, hormone replacement therapy (HRT) attracted much attention. For decades, women had taken HRT to relieve symptoms associated with menopause. Increasing numbers of women, however, were also taking HRT to prevent postmenopausal diseases such as heart disease and osteoporosis. Questions arose. Should women take HRT following a diagnosis of low bone density? Would HRT prevent osteoporosis? Was the hormone therapy linked to an increased risk for breast cancer? There seemed to be many information gaps, and women often joked that they felt between a rock and a hard place, that the choices were too difficult. This book, then, is also for women in general who want information that cuts through much of the anxiety surrounding osteoporosis.

A revelation came in 1999. My son, Jude, was staying in a cabin on a lake in Manitoba, Canada, for a weekend. Among the magazines in the cabin was a 1998 Homemakers magazine with a cover article by journalist Elaine Dewar titled "Breaking News — Blowing the Whistle on Osteoporosis." Jude mailed me the article, which called into question the accuracy of bone density testing diagnoses. The article referred to a large Canadian study that found DXA machines using the manufacturers' reference standards for measuring bone density were diagnosing up to three times as many cases of osteoporosis than when a Canadian reference standard was used. The findings were significant: Osteoporosis had come to be defined by low bone density, though, as the Canadian study discovered, DXA manufacturers had not standardized their machines.

Suddenly I realized that every aspect of the disease was up for debate. Was osteoporosis as prevalent as people were being led to believe? Were people being prescribed medication who were not at risk? Was bone density even an accurate predictor of osteoporosis? If low bone density was not necessarily a cause for concern, why were drugs to increase bone density being prescribed so readily? What did this mean for my parents, my sister, my son and daughter? What did it mean for the millions of women who were being tested and told they had the disease? Why was nobody questioning how osteoporosis had gone from being rare to being everywhere?

> *The more I read, the more convinced I became that women and their doctors were misinformed.*

The more I read, the more I was convinced that women and their doctors were misinformed. I uncovered increasing amounts of evidence that well women were being frightened into unnecessary testing, handed questionable diagnoses, and urged to undergo long-term treatments for a disease that they probably didn't have. I discovered that there are many risk factors for osteoporosis in addition to low bone density, and that when osteoporosis is defined as a condition of fragile bones that fracture easily, it is, in fact, a rare disease. I began to feel hope for my children. Maybe their bones were stronger than I thought.

Then one day I had a major breakthrough. I was spending hours each week in the medical school library searching medical journals, unearthing articles, and following any lead, reference, or footnote that would provide further insight into the disease. One article referred to a 1997 report by the British Columbia Office of Health Technology Assessment. The independent, government-funded agency reviewed evidence to determine the effectiveness of bone mineral density testing. The agency reported that BMD testing does not accurately identify women who will go on to fracture as they age — a finding that prompted a Canadian Broadcasting Corp. documentary that alerted the public to what it called "the marketing of fear" to well women. The report referred to a study that had found that the cracks in Vancouver's sidewalks were a common cause of hip fractures, and that screening large populations of menopausal women for osteoporosis might only prevent between 1 percent and 5 percent of fractures in the elderly. The review raised concerns about overdiagnosis of the disease and overprescribing of medication and addressed the issue of the ineffectiveness of current drug therapies. Similar reviews in countries including the United States, United Kingdom, France, Sweden, and Australia reached the same conclusions — though the results of these government-funded projects rarely rated a mention in the press. The overriding message remained that BMD testing was a reliable and effective way to diagnosis osteoporosis.

My attention moved to the popular treatments for osteoporosis — HRT, bisphosphonates, and the much-heralded prevention strategies of calcium and dairy consumption. There was little evidence to recommend the widely advertised pharmaceuticals or the daily taking of calcium. Coming from a dairy-producing nation that readily accepts the claim that milk consumption results in healthy bones, I was particularly stunned to find that the evidence in favor of dairy just wasn't there. My greatest concern, however, was for the millions of women worldwide who were trustingly taking hormone replacement therapy in the belief that it was protecting their bones. There was minimal evidence that HRT prevented fractures, and there was a growing body of evidence that it caused breast cancer and heart disease.

Then in July 2002, the National Institutes of Health released startling findings from its Women's Health Initiative — one of the largest studies of its kind ever undertaken. Researchers announced that HRT use was linked to an increased risk for breast cancer, heart disease, clotting, and stroke. Doctors' offices and clinics were flooded with calls from worried women who had been taking HRT in the belief that it was keeping them well. Many women stopped HRT and were in great need of information and reassurance.

In the months that followed, I spent many hours talking to women and listening to their stories as part of a national campaign to disseminate accurate information. Some women had been taking HRT for 20 years or more but had no idea why. Others believed HRT to be a wonder drug that would keep them youthful while preventing menopausal discomfort and age-related diseases. Many women felt depressed, fearful, and betrayed. Now, many women had to decide which treatment, if any, to undertake. Osteoporosis-preventing drugs such as alendronate (marketed as Fosamax) and raloxifene (Evista) began to fill the void left by HRT. However, questions remain because long-term safety data on these drugs are limited or nonexistent. Preliminary research also indicates that such treatments provide limited benefit.

I wrote this book to provide current, accurate, and important information. I encourage women to learn the facts about osteoporosis so that they can see through many of the myths surrounding the disease. I encourage women to question the diagnosis of osteoporosis. Most importantly, I encourage women to investigate all of their options for staying well and maintaining excellent bone health.

❊ 2 ❊
The Myth of Risk

Myth #1: Every woman over the age of 50 is at risk for osteoporosis.

At age 45, Ann agreed to have a bone density scan. Her doctor recommended it and emphasized that it was the responsible thing for women her age to do as they approach menopause. As Ann pulled herself off the radiology table after her bone densitometry test, the technician assessing the computerized results warned her that by the time she was 80 she could "be in big trouble." Ann felt shocked and anxious. A follow-up visit to a specialist confirmed that she had "decreased bone density" and included advice that she should immediately begin a calcium supplement program and return for a scan in two years to monitor a potentially serious situation. Her low bone density was blamed on a lifelong aversion to dairy products and two back-to-back pregnancies, followed by lengthy periods of breastfeeding.

Ann is a very fit person with a small build and no family history of osteoporosis. She lacks risk factors for the disease — she doesn't smoke, drink, or take any medications, and she has an excellent diet. She has had no personal history of low-trauma fractures, a sign associated with the disease. Ann does not have osteoporosis. She has osteopenia, or low bone density, and even that diagnosis is questionable given the wide variation of measurements with bone densitometry (DXA) machines.[1] Furthermore, this level of bone density may be normal for her. Labeling her results as "decreased bone density" is puzzling, as the specialist had no prior record of Ann's bone density. More importantly, the test did not tell her about the *strength* of her bones — it is not designed to do that.

There is something deeply disturbing about being told that you have osteoporosis, particularly in the absence of symptoms or disease. It is like hearing that your cherished family home is structurally unsound, that termites have eaten away at the foundation and it could collapse at any time. With your house, you can always move to another building, but when it comes to your body, moving out is not an option. The effect of a diagnosis of osteoporosis can be shattering. People react in different ways. Very little attention has been paid to the psychological impact of such a diagnosis. One study showed that many women stopped exercising, avoided lifting heavy objects, and generally limited physical activity after being told they were at risk for fracture — the very opposite of what is recommended.[2] Others immediately embark upon long-term drug regimens that may carry life-threatening risks, far more serious than a broken wrist bone or a loss of height.[3]

What the specialist should have done was reassure Ann that her bones are probably normal for a small-framed person.[4] He should have told her that bone mineral density (BMD) is only a small part of the osteoporosis story. Lacking other risk factors, her chances of fracturing because of fragile bones were minimal.[5] Had he advised her according to published research, he would have told her that there is no evidence that dairy foods reduce the risk of fracture.[6] In fact, he would have commented that her diet was more than adequate. He could have reassured her that, even though bone density may be lost during pregnancy and lactation, it recovers quickly, regardless of the interval between pregnancies.[7] He should have encouraged her to remain fit and to do weight-bearing exercise. If she wanted to take anything, a balanced bone nutrient supplement is the most he should have recommended. Instead, he has added her to the ever-growing list of "worried well" women who believe themselves candidates for a crippling disease.

Fifty years ago osteoporosis was rare. Doctors considered it an uncommon bone disease, not a women's disease. Until 20 years ago, most of us had never heard of it. Spontaneous fracturing of hips or compressing of vertebrae resulting in painful curvature of the spine was unusual and confined to the very elderly. In

> *Fifty years ago osteoporosis was defined as an uncommon bone disease, not a women's disease.*

contrast, osteoporosis foundations throughout the world are now warning of an epidemic. We are told that one in two Western women (and one in three men) will suffer a bone density related fracture in their lifetime, 20 percent will die within six months of a hip fracture, and another 50 percent will require long-term nursing care.[8] The slogan of the U.S. Osteoporosis Prevention Campaign in May 2001 was "Every 20 Seconds, Osteoporosis Causes a Fracture."[9]

Statistics like these suggest that the disease is more widespread than breast cancer, AIDS, and heart disease combined. How did this happen? More importantly, is it true? If so, surely our hospital beds should be full of people with fractures, and most elderly women should have severely curved spines (dowager's humps).

In addition, osteoporosis foundations predict that there will be a 50 percent increase in the disease in the next 15 years. World elderly populations are growing, consistent with the global population explosion of the last 50 years. It is estimated that 1.7 million hip fractures were suffered by senior citizens in the world in 1990. That number is expected to increase to 6 million by 2050 *based solely on increasing populations and increased life expectancy.* The expanded populations in Asia, Africa, and South America are predicted to lead to massive increases in the numbers of elderly people. Consequently, there is an expected shifting of the "burden of the osteoporosis disease" from the developed world to the developing world, despite the very low rates of fracture in these countries. In 1998, the incidence of hip fracture in mainland China was one of the lowest in the world.[10] Yet, an article on the International Osteoporosis Foundation's Web site estimates that some 212 million fractures will occur annually in China by 2050.[11] Is this truth or fiction?

Osteoporosis

While osteoporosis has been present in human populations for thousands of years, it has always been recorded as affecting only a small fraction of the population. Although there is little recorded evidence of the disease in antiquity, in a rare find, the skeleton of a postmenopausal woman from Lisht, Upper Egypt, dated to the 12th Dynasty (1990–1786 B.C.), has been recently scanned to reveal a hip fracture and compression fractures of some of the vertebrae.[12]

> **Osteoporosis Definitions**
> **Old & New**
>
> **Old Use**
> *Osteoporosis:* A disease where bones fracture as the result of little impact, because they have become thin, brittle, and weak.
>
> **Currently Promoted Use**
> *Osteoporosis:* A condition characterized by low bone mineral density or reduced bone quantity.

Osteoporosis used to be defined as a *disease* where bones fracture as a result of little impact because they have become thin, brittle, and have lost tensile strength. Today, a new definition of osteoporosis has been accepted by the medical community, which defines it as a *condition* characterized by low bone density or reduced bone quantity. This definition says nothing about bone quality — that is, its strength or brittleness. It says very little about the tendency to fracture.

Everybody loses bone density as they age, but the vast majority of the population never fracture as a result of low bone density. The disease osteoporosis is uncommon, even rare, in women under the age of 80. After age 80, most fractures are likely to occur due to other factors involving illness and frailty. These are the factors that predispose someone to falling, such as dementia and medications like sleeping pills and antidepressants. Other factors associated with frailty, such as immobility and malnutrition can further contribute to thinning of bone, as can medications such as corticosteroids. Under these conditions, almost any elderly person may fall and fracture his or her hip. The older and more unwell a person is, the greater the risk of fracture. Simply maintaining a good level of health and fitness will help a well woman in her 50s and 60s to avert such an event.

Osteoporosis is thought of as a disease when in most cases, it is just a condition. People are diagnosed with osteoporosis because they have low bone density, not because they have fractured. This occurs routinely despite the fact that BMD testing does *not* accurately identify women who will go on to fracture.[13] A person with high bone density may fracture, and another with low bone density may never fracture. Low BMD is but one of many risk factors for a disease that can only be truly diagnosed when there is a "fragility" fracture — a fracture resulting from low impact or trauma. Calling low BMD osteoporosis is like calling elevated cholesterol heart disease, or calling high blood pressure a stroke.

When it is characterized by fragile bones that break easily, osteoporosis is a serious, though rare, disease with potentially devastating consequences. But since osteoporosis was redefined as normal age-related bone loss, the worried well now have a new diagnosis. A vast number of supposedly at-risk people are encouraged to take expensive tests and drugs to prevent something that most of them will probably never have.

The vast majority of postmenopausal women need not be concerned about osteoporosis. There is substantial evidence that a good diet, healthy lifestyle, and regular exercise are sufficient protection against future fracture. Many experts agree. Mark Helfand, one of the members of the U.S. National Institutes of Health (NIH) consensus panel on the prevention, diagnosis and treatment of osteoporosis, stated in a Washington Post article: "I think even people who agree that osteoporosis is a serious health problem can still say it is being hyped. It is hyped. Most of what you could do to prevent osteoporosis later in life has nothing to do with getting a test or taking a drug."[14]

Misleading Information

The information from the osteoporosis literature, most doctors, advertising, and the media is misleading and most often inaccurate. These inaccuracies have been allowed to proliferate unchecked without public policy intervention or objective analysis. Challenging evidence has been published repeatedly in prestigious medical journals. Still, the message that predominates is the myth that virtually all women more than 50 years old face the specter of debilitating pain, loss of independence, and immobility. Evidence-based articles contradict many commonly held beliefs about the prevalence, diagnosis, and treatment of osteoporosis. This other side of the story is known to the best osteoporosis specialists and those who stay informed. It has been published in the medical literature, discussed at conferences, yet has somehow failed to filter through to the public. Most ill-informed appear to be the doctors who help "at-risk" patients make decisions regarding their bone health. Too often they base decisions on misinformation, not facts.

A massive osteoporosis-preventing industry has emerged based on the myth of risk. This industry can only increase in size, as more and more of the graying female baby boom population acquire the low bone density "risk factor" for osteoporosis — simply by virtue of their age. Consequently, age is seen as reason enough to perpetuate the idea that hip fracture and subsequent disability are inevitable, unless steps are taken to avoid them.

Promulgating the Myth

In the early 1980s, most women had never heard of osteoporosis, and doctors saw very few patients with the disease. But that was about to change. In 1982, a major promotional campaign sponsored by pharmaceutical companies producing hormone replacement therapy (HRT) set out to create public awareness of osteoporosis as an important women's health issue. The campaign included massive radio, television, and magazine coverage with articles and advertisements published in Vogue, McCall's, and Reader's Digest. Although the campaign focused on the disfigurement of the dowager's hump and the damage of the disease, the companies clearly stood to benefit from increasing public awareness of this condition. Fearful women who went to their doctors to discuss prevention were likely to end up with a prescription for HRT. Yet astoundingly, there was no evidence from placebo-controlled trials that hormone replacement would even prevent or treat osteoporosis.

So successful was the campaign that by the mid-1980s most European and American women had not only heard of the disease, they were increasingly fearful of it. They were convinced of the apparent inevitability of hip fractures and were frightened of becoming like the elderly woman with the severely bent spine seen in calcium advertisements.[15] The medical profession in turn was convinced that osteoporosis was reaching epidemic proportions and that their role was to identify and treat these patients.

In their review of the evidence for the effectiveness of bone mineral density testing, the British Columbia Office of Health Technology Assessment quotes from a report:

> Many advertisements play on the fear of aging, such as the spot for a calcium supplement that shows a healthy 30-year-old women transformed to a stooped 65-year-old in 30 seconds. While such an image capitalizes on the fear of losing youthful beauty, it draws on even deeper fears of disability leading to loss of independence.

> The information on hip fractures is equally frightening. For example, a popular guide to preventing osteoporosis states: "The consequences of osteoporosis can be devastating. Fewer than one-half of all women who suffer a hip fracture regain normal function. Fifteen percent die shortly after their injury, and nearly 30 percent die within a year." The fear for women is that even if they survive a hip fracture, they may face long years of dependency and immobility.[16]

The advertisements fail to mention that the majority of postmenopausal women who do have spinal (vertebral) fractures are unaware of the fact and have no symptoms. They also ignore the fact that most fractures occur only in the very elderly and are linked to many other complicating factors. The truth is that most women who suffer hip fractures are aged 85 or older and are unwell. Many of the women who did not recover had been in declining health preceding their fractures. While a hip fracture was part of the disability surrounding their deaths, it did not cause them. It is estimated that as few as 14 percent of deaths following a hip or pelvic fracture were caused or hastened by the fracture in women who were walking and active prior to the event.[17]

> *Most fractures occur due to complicating factors other than low bone density, and most women who have vertebral (spinal) fractures have no symptoms.*

Advertisements, media campaigns, and fact sheets in doctors' waiting rooms grossly exaggerate the numbers of people who fracture and the impact that osteoporosis can have on a postmenopausal woman's life.

The Redefining of Osteoporosis

In 1994, in the wake of the globally successful osteoporosis marketing campaign, a new definition of osteoporosis was created that was so broad that it would diagnose half of all postmenopausal women as diseased. Osteoporosis had previously been characterized by fragility fractures — that is, bones breaking under relatively low impact. Examples of fragility fractures include falling off a chair, tripping while walking, or stubbing your toe with resultant fracture. In contrast, high-impact trauma is when you fracture your leg in a skiing accident, or your ribs in a car accident. High-impact trauma represents conditions under which any bone would break.

In 1988, Dual X-ray Absorptiometry (DXA) machinery was developed to measure the bone mineral density (BMD) of an individual to determine the likelihood that a person will develop osteoporosis. DXA has become the internationally recognized

> *Bone mineral density testing measures only bone mass, not the factors that contribute to bone fragility, such as bone size, shape, and internal support (trabecular cross-bracing).*

gold standard for determining osteoporosis risk. But BMD only measures bone mass, not the factors which contribute to bone fragility, such as bone size and shape, vertebral body diameter, hip axis length and loss of trabecular cross-bracing.

Bone mineral density naturally decreases with age in most people, but not all people are at risk for fragility fractures. The impressive development of sophisticated DXA technology had created the potential for measuring low BMD. This allowed low bone mineral density to take a quantum leap from the category of a hidden risk factor to the category of an easily diagnosed disease.

In 1994, a World Health Organization (WHO) committee of experts established an international standard which now gives a bone

> ### Bone Density Testing Categories
>
> **Normal:** A value for bone mineral density or content within 1 standard deviation (SD) of the young adult reference mean.
>
> **Osteopenia:** A value for bone mineral density or content more than 1 SD below the young adult mean but less than 2.5 SD below this value.
>
> **Osteoporosis:** A value for bone mineral density or content 2.5 SD or more below the young adult mean.
>
> **Severe (Established) Osteoporosis:** A value for bone mineral density or content 2.5 SD or more below the young adult mean in the presence of one or more fragility fractures.

mineral density reading 2.5 standard deviations below "normal" a diagnosis of *osteoporosis*. Readings 1.0 to 2.5 standard deviations below normal are classified as *osteopenia*, or low bone density — the early stage of osteoporosis. The normal level is currently determined by an assumed average peak bone density of young white women. This is known as a T-score. For each standard deviation decrease in bone mineral density, doctors are warned that fracture risk in their patient is predicted to double.[18] This means that unless women maintain their bone mass at peak levels throughout their life span, they will be labeled at risk or diseased. The natural biological variation among healthy adults and the normal age-related bone loss are not accounted for by this definition. Neither is the all-important fact that low bone density is not a good predictor of future fracture.

This new definition meant that millions of women suddenly qualified for diagnosis of a disease for which they had never considered themselves at risk. As one expert in osteoporosis recently put it: "If you want to make more people have osteoporosis, simply change the definition of osteoporosis or use a kind of bone density measurement that decreases with age [i.e., the T-Score]."[19]

Both these things have happened. The definition of osteoporosis has changed from fragility fractures to a measure of bone density. The "normal" level is a young person with high bone density. That ensures that age-related decrease in bone density is automatically categorized as abnormal.

The impact of the redefining of osteoporosis is considerable. Once a woman has been diagnosed as having low bone density, she is often hooked into a lifetime of screening, monitoring, and drug therapy. Based in large part on this redefinition, some 37 percent (16 million) of all U.S. postmenopausal women were using HRT (hormone replacement therapy) by 1999, and by 2000, HRT had become the No. 1 prescription drug in the world.[20,21] The numbers of women on HRT remain at almost 10 million in 2003, despite the Women's Health Initiative Study demonstrating that long-term use of HRT is not safe.[22]

One assumes that the World Health Organization is an independent and neutral body, untainted by any conflict of interest in its assessments and reports. But the WHO study group on bone densitometry screening that defined the thresholds for diagnosing osteoporosis was funded by three major drug companies.[23] From this initial meeting emerged similarly funded conferences worldwide. Despite widespread criticism, this new definition has been adopted as the mainstream measure for diagnosing osteoporosis.

Today many international independent review groups do not sanction the WHO definition, and many have argued against its use. The Swedish Council on Technology Assessment in Health Care demonstrated that the WHO's use of healthy young women as a reference group resulted in large numbers of women being wrongly defined as abnormal. Using the WHO standards, they estimate that 22 percent of all women over the age of 50 will be defined as having osteoporosis, and 52 percent as having osteopenia. The Swedish council also raised concerns that "defining a complex, often lifelong, process such as osteoporosis in terms of a single BMD measurement is highly problematic and should be critically examined."[24]

Despite concerns, the definition has been widely accepted by the scientific community. The flaws in such a simple definition are many:

> *Peak bone mass is virtually indefinable, as it varies from race to race, between genders, seasons, and even geographical regions of a country.*

I. It assumes that bone density predicts a person's future risk of fracture. It has not been shown conclusively that it can. It assumes that the young reference peak bone mass used in the DXA machine assessment is an accurate representation of everyone's peak bone mass (gained in early adulthood). Peak bone mass, though, is virtually indefinable, as it varies from race to race, between genders, across geographical regions of a country, and even between seasons. In 1998, Dr. Alan Tenenhouse, the principal investigator of a groundbreaking Canadian study, revealed that "the most interesting thing we've learned is that peak bone mass varies across the country ... We can't find any real differences to explain it. It's substantial. The difference is greater than 10 percent, which is more than one DXA standard deviation."[25]

2. Most alarmingly, there is no international normal reference standard for DXA machines. Manufacturers set their own, often high standards, resulting in widely varying diagnoses. Results will vary between machines, regions, and countries.

3. The criteria only apply to Caucasian women. It is known that a huge variation in bone mass exists between ethnic groups, and between men and women. A study of four ethnic groups — Hawaiian, Filipino, Japanese, and Caucasian women — found differences in peak bone mass varying up to 100 percent.[26] It is essential, therefore, that a reference standard based on a local population of the same ethnicity be used when measuring bone density — something that is rarely done.

The WHO definition was apparently designed to convince policymakers of the perceived magnitude of the osteoporosis problem.[27] It was clearly successful. It has since netted far more of the population than was ever anticipated (or predicted by the standard definition model). This is certainly cause to question such an arbitrary definition. But the osteoporosis societies of the United States and other Western countries now routinely state that 50 percent of all women over the age of 50 are at risk for osteoporosis. They continue to propagate the myth that all women over the age of 50 are at risk for this disease.

What About Fracture Rates?

All this is ignoring one essential factor — the presence of fracture. Because the real concern is breaking bones, the preoccupation with measuring bone mineral density tends to eclipse this obvious and important indicator. You may have low bone density and never fracture; or you may have normal bone density and fracture. Although it is repeatedly overlooked in the publicized WHO definition of osteoporosis, "established osteoporosis" is defined by low BMD *along with one or more fractures resulting from low impact or trauma.*

> *The fact is that you may have low bone density and never fracture. Or you may have normal or better than normal bone density and still have a fracture.*

When determining the incidence of osteoporosis, low bone density is not being distinguished from established osteoporosis, which is defined by the prevalence of fractures. This creates enormous confusion when trying to make sense of osteoporosis statistics, because in most cases, they are based on BMD alone, not fracture rates.

The bone mineral density definition of osteoporosis has contributed to the medicalization of aging women, based on a technology that science has yet to prove is effective. The British Columbia Office of Health Technology Assessment review of the evidence for the effectiveness of bone mineral density testing concludes: "BMD testing is unable to accurately distinguish women at low risk of fracture from those at high risk."[28]

A Caucasian woman's estimated likelihood of an osteoporosis-related fracture after age 50 will depend on the country of residence, the information source, the disease definition, and the interpretation of fracture data. It will range from 10 percent to 56 percent. Most estimates are in the 50 percent range, but fail to explain that this is based on:

- Wrist (or Colles') fractures which tend to happen to women in their 60s and 70s, and may or may not be linked to osteoporosis. There is little evidence that BMD plays a part in these fractures, as DXA measurement of the forearm does not seem to be able to predict them. A Colles' fracture can occur with normal, high, or low bone density of the forearm.[29]

> **About Vertebral Fractures**
>
> According to Dr. Bruce Ettinger, Senior Investigator, Division of Research, Kaiser Permanente Medical Care Program, California, "Only 5 percent to 7 percent of 70-year-olds will show vertebral collapse; only half of these will have two involved vertebrae; and perhaps one-fifth or one-sixth will have symptoms. I have a very big practice and I have very few bent-over patients. There's been a tremendous hullabaloo lately, and there are a lot of worried women — and excessive testing and administration of medications."(Medical Review, 1985)[30]

- A loose and hotly debated definition of vertebral "fractures." Most vertebral fractures result in loss of height without any major symptoms. No comparison can be made between the seriousness of hip fractures versus vertebral fractures.

- Hip fractures that occur between the age of 80 and 90 are invariably linked to factors other than osteoporosis. Many elderly people suffer from poor eyesight and other serious medical problems like dementia. Many in this age group are on several prescription medications that can trigger falls and fractures, including corticosteroids, powerful long-acting tranquilizers, and antipsychotics. Falling and breaking a hip, therefore, is most often a marker of generally frail health. In most cases, it has little to do with osteoporosis.[31] In fact, falling in a particular way will fracture the neck of the femur, regardless of bone strength or density. A man or woman who remains fit and well is less likely to fracture.

- A 50-year-old women has only a 15 percent chance of a hip fracture by the time she is 80. Only a small percentage of that 15 percent will have life-threatening complications from the fracture.

When these factors are taken into account, it is clear that the risk of an osteoporosis-related fracture is nothing near 50 percent. Dr. Bruce Ettinger reassures further: "Women shouldn't worry about osteoporosis. The osteoporosis that causes pain and disability is a very rare disease."[32] Despite this, the media and doctors continue to warn middle-aged women that they must act now to avert a life-threatening disease that can bring death, disability, deformity, and loss of independence.

The absence of internationally agreed-upon criteria for measuring fracture statistics and the debate surrounding the redefinition of osteoporosis as a condition of low bone density has led to widely diverging statistics concerning osteoporosis and osteoporosis-related fractures:

- The Mayo Clinic: In the United States, about 21 percent of postmenopausal women have osteoporosis and about 16 percent have had a fracture.[33]

- U.S. National Osteoporosis Foundation: One in two women and one in eight men over age 50 will have an osteoporosis-related fracture in their lifetime.[34]

- The Canadian Multi-Centered Osteoporosis Study (2000): In Canada, approximately 16 percent of women and 5 percent of men suffer from osteoporosis.[35]

- National Health and Nutrition Examination Survey III: The age-adjusted prevalence of osteoporosis in women aged 50 years and older was 21 percent in European-Americans, compared to 16 percent for Mexican-Americans and 10 percent for African-Americans.[36]

- International Osteoporosis Foundation: Worldwide, the lifetime risk for a woman to have an osteoporotic fracture is 30 percent to 40 percent. In men, the risk is about 13 percent.[37]

- National Osteoporosis Society UK: 1 in 3 women and at least 1 in 12 men will develop osteoporosis during their lifetime.[38]

- Australian Osteoporosis Society: It is estimated that the proportion of women with osteoporosis increases from 15 percent in those aged 60 to 64 years up to 71 percent in those more than 80 years of age. The incidence is much lower in men, ranging from 1.6 percent of those aged 60 to 64 years to 19 percent of those aged more than 80 years.[39]

- Osteoporosis New Zealand: Osteoporosis is a major health issue with 56 percent of all postmenopausal women predicted to have an osteoporosis-related fracture.[40]

- Professor Ian Reid, from the Auckland Medical School, New Zealand: "People might be surprised to know that everyone has osteoporosis, though most to a lesser extent. No one is immune to it really. It is a condition we all have after 40."[41]

Statements on the incidence of fracture are constructed from data that is open to wide interpretation. Dr. Susan Ott, Associate Professor of Medicine, University of Washington, an international osteoporosis authority, comments:

> Counting the actual number of fractures related to osteoporosis is more difficult than it appears and requires strict criteria. It would be quite easy to make the figures high if you wanted. Obviously, a huge number of people fracture as the result of accidents, and who says how many of those should be counted? What actually constitutes a fracture of spinal vertebrae is also dependent upon how the vertebrae are measured. Loss of height has been used as a measure and when a small amount of height loss is applied then fracture rates are very high. However, when stricter criteria involving spinal X-rays and measurement of vertebrae are involved there are far fewer fractures.[42]

How do you decide? Dr. R. P. Heaney, osteoporosis expert, writes:

> Any bone will break if pressure is applied in a particular way, so falling patterns are also a big factor. Even young normal bone will fracture if struck just so; many elderly fragility fractures are of precisely this sort.[43]

Times Have Changed

It is simply not possible to assume that women currently turning 50 will have the same rate of fracture as women who are in the high-risk elderly age group. Those women who are aged 75 to 100 now were born between 1903 and 1926. Their peak bone mass was being developed up until the end of World War II — a period which spanned the Great Depression and two world wars with the associated poverty, compromised nutrition, and disrupted lifestyles. Who can say that women currently entering menopause are going to have the same fracture rates as their mothers and grandmothers? Chances are they will be very different. This is particularly so, given dietary and lifestyle changes, and the control the baby boomers have had over reproduction, with fewer pregnancies and greater numbers of menstrual periods. Circulating ovarian hormone levels are very different in the woman who is repeatedly pregnant and lactating, and it is well known that reproductive hormones influence bone metabolism. Whether this influences bone health for the better however, is unknown, as is the effect of long-term exposure to synthetic hormones in the form of the oral contraceptive pill, HRT, and environmental hormone-mimicking chemicals.

Women and Aging

Aging in the West is about losses, not gains, and Western clinical medicine has been very influenced by popular perceptions of women and aging. Younger women of reproductive age are considered the standard for what is normal and healthy, and aging women are often considered in terms of hormone deficiency, a condition that needs to be treated with hormone supplements. Reputed to replace the now "missing" hormones, HRT had been heralded as the panacea for the aging woman. It promised to deal with menopause discomfort while simultaneously halting age-related bone loss, and by definition, osteoporosis.

The onset of menopause is equated not just with loss of fertility, but also loss of youth, femininity, sexual desirability, and social status. Ours is not a society that tends to place value on life experience and wisdom — thus older women can experience a sense of social redundancy. They often feel a deep fear of disability and the loss of independence.

Magazine articles and books on menopause tend to emphasize the biological changes that occur and perpetuate the idea that the aging female body is in a state of decline. Biological changes associated with aging are discussed in the language of abnormality and decay. Terms such as "failing ovaries" and "estrogen deficiency" label the aging woman as a diseased woman. So entrenched is the idea that the older woman is somehow diseased, that many women expect their minds and bodies to deteriorate after menopause.

In the British Columbia Office of Health Technology Assessment's (BCOHTA) review of the evidence for selective BMD testing in Canada, the authors make this point:

> The effects of medicalization on a social group can be far-reaching and subtle. For example, as natural phenomena become labeled as disease, anxiety is heightened. The general public is inundated about the "discov-

ered" disease. Social science research of medicine has repeatedly demonstrated how market forces may capitalize on a climate of risk and reassurance, which then drives the use of health technologies regardless of whether they lead to improved health outcome. This has been shown for ultrasound, electronic fetal monitors, predictive genetic screening, and mammography, among others.[44]

There is the psychology that if aging is a disease, then it is a potentially curable one. The physician is expected to offer regular screening to monitor the signs of decline and to prescribe treatment to avert diseases.

An associated BCOHTA article puts bone mineral density testing in its social context:

> Once the fear of becoming diseased has been created, women are made to feel personally accountable for managing their risk of disease and future illness, and are encouraged to take appropriate measures to prevent it. Given that menopause has been defined in terms of hormone deficiency and osteoporosis increasingly defined in relation to that deficiency, any woman who wishes to avoid the "diseases" of aging will have to be tested for BMD and, if deficient, will have to embark on HRT.
>
> … Individuals taking up this burden of preventing sickness and striving more and more to reach the ideal of normality may struggle in vain. The proliferation of disease categories and labels in medicine and psychiatry results in even more restricted definitions of "normal." This leads to increasing numbers of people being labeled abnormal, sick, or deviant. The area of "normality" is shrinking and the area of "abnormality" or less than perfect health is increasing.[45]

Research of other cultures indicates that the menopause-associated decline is a uniquely Western phenomenon. In many cultures, the arrival of menopause signals a new freedom. It is associated with an increased social status where women gain worth and veneration. The cultural expectation to live a long and healthy life can be self-fulfilling. Individuals who integrate that expectation do live longer. In traditional Japanese society, for example, women expect to continue to be well. They become respected elders and fulfill a valued role in their communities. Anthropologists also note that menopause passes by unmarked socially or biologically in some cultures. This is particularly so where frequent pregnancy and lactation is the norm. In these cultures, cessation of menstruation is relatively unremarkable.[46]

Osteoporosis and Aging

Many countries have not identified osteoporosis as a disease to be concerned about. Rates of fracture are very low in Africa, South America, and most of Asia. In countries like Cambodia, it is reported to be unheard of.[47]

Gradual loss of bone density occurs naturally in all males and females with aging, and at varying rates with different bone sites. Some bones actually gain density with age, and others lose very little mass. Age-related bone density loss does not as a matter of course equate with fragility fractures.

The deeply entrenched idea that osteoporosis is reaching epidemic proportions makes it difficult for anyone to seriously challenge the status quo. Women assume that their doctors are fully informed about the prevalence, diagnosis, and treatment of osteoporosis. Virtually no one questions the appropriateness of widespread DXA screening, or the impact of a diagnosis of low bone density on a well woman. The unsuspecting patient and well-intentioned doctor are unaware in most cases that DXA screening is inaccurate and not a good predictor of fracture risk. They simply do not know that front-line therapies for treating osteoporosis have serious associated risks and limited evidence to support their effectiveness in preventing fracture.

Women are easily swayed because the medicalization of menopause has paved the way for the medicalization of bone mineral loss. Women have not questioned this because of the public perception that modern medicine and technology hold the answers to eliminating health risks. But maybe it is time for us to rethink this. An article in the Journal of the American Medical Association confirmed that doctors are the third-leading cause of death in the United States, after cancer and heart disease. Every year, 250,000 deaths result from medication errors, errors in hospitals, unnecessary surgery, and the negative effects of drugs. The author of the article, Barbara Starfield, puts the figures in context: Prescription drugs alone claim 106,000 lives annually in the United States. That is equivalent to three jumbo-jet crashes every two days.[48]

> *Over 106,000 deaths occur annually in the United States due to prescription drugs, taken as directed, without error in dosing.*

Women in Western countries have accepted they are at risk for a disease, purely by virtue of their gender and reproductive status. Yet, the evidence that every aspect of the disease is controversial is found throughout the medical literature. The concept that all women over the age of 50 are at risk for osteoporosis is a myth.

✵ 3 ✵

The Myth of Diagnosis

Myth #2: Diagnosis of osteoporosis is accurate,
reliable, and meaningful.

Doubtful Diagnoses

The accuracy and precision of bone density testing and its validity as a means to diagnose osteoporosis is increasingly controversial. In October 2001, a New Zealand "20/20" television documentary examined the issues surrounding osteoporosis. In a simple experiment, the producers sent Sally, a healthy, 50-year-old woman, to be scanned by two different major brands of DXA machines in separate cities. In an outcome that stunned viewers, she was only fractionally below normal on one DXA machine, but on the other had bone density so low that it was close to the threshold for a diagnosis of osteoporosis. In one clinic, she was given a clean bill of health, and in the other, she was advised to undergo treatment.

Osteoporosis is a complex condition that is still not fully understood. Diagnosis is, therefore, not as simple as it may appear. A diagnosis of established osteoporosis can only really be made once there has been a fracture as the result of low impact or low trauma, which is confirmation that bone fragility exists. In the absence of fractures, osteoporosis is invisible and painless, and there is currently no way to accurately predict who will fracture.

Bone density measurement is a modern phenomenon. We have no idea what the bone densities of our parents or grandparents were as they grew up, or even what our own were as children. Thus, it is difficult to define what is normal during the stages of a given person's lifetime. Because most studies have only measured changes over short periods, and accurate methods for testing bone mineral density have only recently become available, there remains a large gap in understanding bone formation and maintenance over a person's life span. With the availability of bone scanning technology, we are able to measure the bone density of young people as it increases to peak bone mass in young adulthood. But this raises many questions about current understandings of what is normal. Based on the World Health Organization (WHO) definition of osteoporosis, only 84 percent of young women in America are reaching normal levels of bone density.[1]

The 1994 WHO definition, which characterizes osteoporosis as a measure of bone mineral density (BMD), has been adopted throughout the world because BMD is the easiest of the osteoporosis risk factors to measure. Bone mineral density has thus become the default definition of osteoporosis. This means, in effect, that one of the many risk factors has become the disease. Consequently, all research, treatment, and preventative approaches are focused on BMD. Screening and diagnosing of healthy women based on BMD continues to increase, despite widespread discrediting of its ability to predict fracture.

Now doctors can assume responsibility for monitoring and managing the density of their patients' bones from the first DXA scan until the end of their lives. The availability of DXA technology has allowed physicians to begin to identify variations in bone mineral density among populations and to observe changes in an individual over time. These observations are of limited value, though, if they don't help to prevent fragility fractures and reduce the incidence of established osteoporosis. Doctors have the dilemma of determining whether low bone density puts their patient at risk, and whether they should be treated.

The review of the effectiveness of BMD testing by the British Columbia Health Technology Assessment Agency (BCOHTA) warns:

> A program which exposes a large segment of the population to lifelong medical attempts to maximize BMD should be required to justify these strategies on the basis of research evidence demonstrating that medical management can alter the natural history of fragility fractures ...

> Even the most favorable reports on the effectiveness of bone mineral testing reveal that BMD testing does *not* accurately identify women who will go on to fracture as they age.[2]

Bone Density — Only Part of the Story

The World Health Organization describes osteoporosis as "a progressive systemic skeletal disease, characterized by low bone mass and micro-architectural deterioration of bone tissue, with a consequent increase in bone fragility and susceptibility to fracture."[3]

This definition identifies two main risk factors — loss of bone quantity and loss of bone quality. DXA scanning measures only bone quantity (bone density or mass), not bone strength. Bone strength is determined by its micro-architecture: its size, shape, trabecular cross-bracing, and ability to repair damage. But, because of difficulties in measuring micro-architecture, that important aspect of bone health has been ignored. Bone density alone has become the focus of research and the definition of osteoporosis.

R.P. Heaney, an international expert on osteoporosis, states:

> The current prominence of BMD is due to the fact that it can be accurately measured and to some extent controlled. Indeed, essentially all preventative and therapeutic approaches to osteoporosis focus explicitly on acquiring and maintaining bone mass or on restoring lost mass. However, low bone mass probably accounts for less than half of all osteoporotic fractures. Thus history of fracture after age 40 and maternal history of hip fracture are stronger predictors than BMD and are independent of BMD.[4]

Indeed, a BMD measurement reveals no information about bone micro-architecture — a DXA scan or an X-ray cannot measure a person's bone quality or strength. At this point, we do not have the technology to estimate bone strength. Therefore, a person may be low in bone mass, but have perfectly normal bone structure and strength.

With severe osteoporosis, the meshed, inter-linked trabecular bone can erode, greatly weakening the bone. But a DXA scan is not able to identify this type of damage. Typically, osteoporosis literature includes pictures of the various stages of osteoporosis. It shows, as the disease progresses, the increasingly fragile and space-filled lacy network of disconnected trabecular bone. The picture looks as though the bone would disintegrate with the slightest of knocks. These are not images from a DXA scan. The images do not relate to diagnoses of osteopenia and osteoporosis. In reality, these familiar images are taken from biopsies or autopsies of older people, not from women with DXA diagnoses of low bone density.

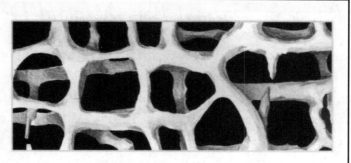

Image of Weakened, Fragile Osteoporotic Bone—Not Identifiable by DXA Scan

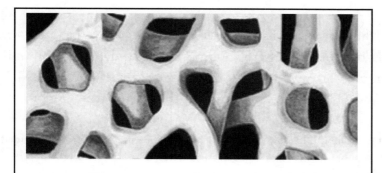

Microscopic Image of Normal Trabecular Bone

Susan Ott, M.D., comments:

Bone quality is determined by bone mass (as measured by bone density) and also by the micro-architecture of bone, the crystal size and shape, the brittleness, the connectivity of the trabecular network, the vitality of the bone cells, ability to repair micro-cracks, and the structure of the bone proteins. The fat cells, vasculature, neuronal pathways, and bone marrow cells probably also influence the quality of the bone as well as the quantity of bone.[5]

The Range of Normal Bone Mineral Density

Significant and unexplained racial differences exist in both bone mass and the prevalence of fractures. If low bone mass is linked to fracture, then we would expect to see more fractures in ethnic groups that have naturally low bone density. This is not the case. While it is true that people of African descent have higher bone mass and lower rates of fractures, it is also true that Asian women have lower bone mass than Caucasian women, without a proportionally higher rate of hip fractures. Hispanic women have approximately half as many fractures as Caucasian women, but their bone density is no different.[6]

In Malmo, Sweden, there is a very high rate of hip fracture — much higher than other Western countries. But a study of the bone mineral density of this population found little evidence that low BMD was the cause. The authors of a study of this phenomenon reported:

> The Malmo bone mineral content was on the same level as in the United States, but higher than in Japan and France. The comparatively high level of fragility fractures in the Scandinavian countries cannot be explained by low bone mass.[7]

Falling is the big problem with the elderly, not bone density. Because any bone will fracture under certain conditions, a review of 28 studies concluded that most elderly women would fracture with the impact of an unprotected fall. The authors stated:

> Differences in bone density between individual women are not great enough to discriminate between who will and who will not later suffer a fracture; this will be determined by chance, by conditions that increase the risk of falling or cause loss of the normal protective reflexes, and by illness and immobility causing bone loss shortly before the fracture.[8]

A similar consideration of the role of BMD testing in identifying vertebral fractures led to this conclusion:

Our knowledge of the incidence and natural course of vertebral fractures and the effectiveness of preventive measures is limited, and with this uncertainty screening for vertebral body fractures cannot at present be recommended.[9]

Measuring a man's BMD using DXA scanning is also problematic. Applying the same standard of peak bone mass to the male skeleton, as is done for females, is probably inappropriate. Men generally have taller and larger skeletons than women. Because DXA adjusts for the area scanned, but doesn't completely correct for the fact that wider bones are also thicker, bigger bones appear to have greater BMD, even if the actual tissue density of bone is no different.[10]

Furthermore, the more elderly the person, the more difficult it is to accurately measure bone density. Many experts agree that measuring bone mineral density of lumbar spine in the elderly, particularly men, is next to useless. This is because compression fractures, arthritis, and other factors create artificially dense bone in the vertebrae of elderly people.

> *Because of arthritis and other factors, measuring the bone mineral density of the lumbar spine in the elderly is next to useless.*

Bone Densitometry Testing

In 1988, Dual X-ray Absorptiometry (DXA) machinery was developed and quickly became the accepted gold standard to measure bone mineral density (BMD) because of its speed, safety, and perceived accuracy. DXA is sophisticated computerized technology that can, in a matter of minutes and with minimal radiation exposure, measure the mineral content of the vertebrae, the hip, the forearm, or even the whole skeleton. It prints out an impressive computer graphic of the bones and reports where a patient's bone mass falls in relation to the "normal" population. DXA measures the bone mineral content (BMC), then divides that by the surface area of the bone being measured to create a bone mineral density (BMD) measurement expressed in terms of grams per square centimeter. This has limitations, as it provides only a two-dimensional reading, not a three-dimensional measurement, as many doctors believe.

The World Health Organization definition finds bone mineral density and bone mineral content equal, or independently reliable, in predicting osteoporosis. But the prevalence of osteoporosis depends entirely upon the way in which DXA results are interpreted and expressed. For example, a United Kingdom study found that the prevalence of osteoporosis of the spine in women more than 70 years old has been found to be approximately 30 percent when measured in terms of BMD, but is only half that when BMC is used.[11]

Dr. S. Pors Neilson discusses this in his article "The fallacy of BMD: a critical review of the diagnostic use of dual X-ray absorptiometry":

> This fact is well-known but is largely neglected. This neglect has the obvious consequence that osteoporosis is overdiagnosed in persons of petite body stature, simply because the means of reference populations are calculated from the values of large and small people.[12]

In addition, the technical accuracy and precision of BMD measurements are considered by some to be barely satisfactory for clinical use. An accurate measurement would represent the true mineral content of the targeted bone site. But the error for DXA measurements can be up to 8 percent. This means that the true value of a woman's bone density could be 8 percent higher or lower than what is reported to her. That is equal to almost one standard deviation, enough to dramatically change her diagnosis.[13]

Precision refers to whether the same bone site can be measured repeatedly with an identical outcome. In the absence of international standards, DXA machines are calibrated differently, so precision is far from guaranteed. For this reason it is important to always be measured using the same machine, using the same reference ranges, in follow-up testing.

> *Because DXA machines are calibrated differently, it is important that follow-up testing be done on the same machine.*

Quantitative Ultrasound

Quantitative ultrasound offers a cheaper, more accessible method of bone density testing. It uses sound waves rather than X-rays, and most commonly measures the calcaneous or heel bone, as it is limited to bone with minimal overlying tissue. It is considered a reasonably useful diagnostic tool, but the results cannot be directly compared with the results of a DXA scan, which remains the industry standard. It is not fully understood exactly what is being measured with heel ultrasound. It appears to mainly measure bone density. A recent study of 149,524 postmenopausal women suggests that ultrasound and peripheral BMD testing may predict an increased risk for fracture. The study found that low BMD in the heel, forearm, or finger measured was associated with a two-fold increased risk for fracture within one year.[14] Still, this method of measuring bone density suffers from the same problems of classification that DXA scanning does — it classifies a large number of women at risk, many of whom will never experience a fracture.

Establishing Normal Peak Bone Mass

DXA measures the bone mineral density of an individual and then "grades" it against an average peak bone mass, or peak bone density, which has been established from a selected young reference population. But as researchers are finding, peak bone mass varies widely from region to region, by gender, and even fluctuates seasonally. A Mexican survey of more than 4,000 healthy young people showed wide regional variations in peak bone density, and a recent Canadian study revealed similar inconsistencies.[15] Consequently, concerned scientists and osteoporosis experts are warning that the technology may be diagnosing "low bone density" when it is at a normal level for that person — a level that may never result in a fracture.

Peak Bone Mass Defined

Adolescence is a crucial time for bone development. Surges in growth and reproductive hormones initiate a spurt in bone growth that is responsible for almost half of the adult bone mass. Peak bone mass (PBM) usually occurs around age 20. It is the total bone mass or density that a young person has after they have completed the growth of their long bones. The level of peak bone mass achieved in any individual is the result of all the things that have happened to the skeleton from its formation in the uterus through the years of growth into young adulthood. It is the sum of genetic and environmental factors. Once peak bone mass is achieved, bone mass tends to remain stable in both males and females until their late 30s and 40s. After this time, it begins to decline, at different rates for different individuals, and at different rates for different sites in the body. Bone density is, on average, lower in women than in men, but there is a wide range among individuals. Women on average lose between one-third and one-half of their peak bone mass over their lifetime, while men lose less.[16]

It is believed that genetic factors account for an estimated 60 percent to 80 percent of the variability in PBM, with diet, physical activity, and hormonal status being important factors as well.[17] Some bones will continue to grow. The skull increases in mass throughout life. Certain bones, the femur (thighbone) and vertebrae, for example, continue to increase in diameter as we get older. It is generally agreed that the greater the peak bone mass achieved in youth, the greater protection a person has against fracture later in life when bone density progressively decreases for everyone. But this is only an assumption and doesn't account for normal variations in PBM and bone density. The natural history of bone development before menopause and changes over a lifetime are particularly poorly understood because of a lack of longitudinal studies with good methodology and design.

Bone Physiology

In general, bone physiology is considered similar in males and females. Structurally, bone is of two types — trabecular bone and cortical bone. Trabecular bone is the more porous, honeycomb-like bone that forms the inner meshwork of the vertebrae, pelvis, flat bones and the ends of long bones. Trabecular bone constitutes 20 percent of the skeleton but has a large surface area and is sensitive to metabolic changes. Trabecular bone is the type of bone most subject to loss of density as we grow older, and to loss of structural integrity and strength with established osteoporosis.

Cortical, or compact bone, which makes up 80 percent of the skeleton, forms the outer casing of all bones and is the major constituent of the shaft of long bones. The loss of bone that occurs with aging results in up to 35 percent reduction of cortical bone and a 50 percent reduction of trabecular bone in women. Men lose approximately 25 percent and 35 percent of cortical and trabecular bone respectively. Interestingly, one study showed that males have larger bones, but not necessarily stronger bones. The trabecular bone density was the same in males and females, and decreased with age in both. Whether DXA scanning using women's criteria for diagnosis is relevant for men is under debate. Generally, the criteria established for women are applied in the same way to men.

Manufacturers' Reference Standards

When you have your bone density measured by a DXA machine, you are given a computerized analysis indicating whether your bone density is normal, above, or below normal. "Normal" is a level set in the software of the DXA machine. If you are more than one standard deviation below that, then you are classified as abnormal.

What most people don't realize is that they are not being compared to their own peak bone mass or to their own age group's. Instead, they are being measured against that of a selected group of young "normal individuals," which has been established by the DXA manufacturer. The WHO definition of osteoporosis recommends all women be measured and diagnosed using a young normal reference population. This is called a T-score. A Z-score is when you are measured against an average BMD for your age and gender, but this is not used to formally diagnose. Because everyone loses bone density as they age, using T-scores instead of Z-scores guarantees that almost all older women will fall into the "negative" range. Their normal age-related bone loss will automatically be categorized as osteopenia or osteoporosis. If Z-scores were used, it is unlikely there would be an epidemic of osteoporosis.

Here is the surprising thing:

There is no agreed international reference standard, and each manufacturer has established its own independent, average young normal data, resulting in vastly different standards between brands of DXA machines.

> *Using T-scores instead of Z-scores guarantees that almost all older women will fall into the 'negative' range.*

The major manufacturers of DXA machines in the United States have created their young normal reference standards by measuring the peak bone mass of healthy, young white women of different ages. For one group, the age range was 20 to 29. For another, it was 20 to 39. One population included women up to the age of 50 years. One manufacturer reported that its reference data was obtained from 3,000 U.S. and Northern European females, 1,400 French females, and 1,400 Japanese females,[18] while another drew its reference subjects from the University of California in San Diego. This latter population is not believed to be a random sample of the population — they were chosen because they were *exceptionally* healthy, so they do not represent a normal, young, healthy adult. Screening in this way can create an artificially high "normal" or mean peak bone mass, which inevitably leads to biased results. Under these conditions, many more people will be found to have low bone density and will consequently be given a diagnosis of osteoporosis.[19]

During the course of their research, the authors of the British Columbia Technology Assessment review of the effectiveness of BMD testing contacted the manufacturers of DXA machines to find out how the "young normal" subjects were selected. Other than obvious reasons for exclusion, such as medication, substance abuse, and illness, they were given very little information about important factors like age, nutrition, exercise patterns, and even weight and height of the individuals. The authors of the study conclude: "We have no assurance that the range of 'young normals' were not biased by the inclusion of a disproportionately large number of athletic team members."[20]

More recently, concerned researchers in various countries have established their own young normal standards based on local populations. They have invariably found them to be different from the manufacturer's — usually much lower. When they have applied their own local reference standards for general screening instead of the manufacturer's, the outcomes have been very different. This suggests that massive variations in diagnosis are taking place — dependent entirely upon which country or which machine is doing the measuring.

Two large studies, one in the United States and one in Canada, measured local population samples of young people in order to set their own DXA reference standards. The studies then measured a large cross section of the population using their local standards and compared this with the manufacturer's standard.

The first study, the third National Health and Nutrition Examination Survey (NHANES III), chose a sample of young women who were more diverse in terms of body size and other environmental factors than the manufacturer's group. For example, young women with pre-existing illnesses who were taking medications were not excluded, and although this was unlikely to affect bone loss, it meant that there was more variation in height and weight than in the healthy volunteers used by the manufacturers. Researchers did this to obtain a reference group that accurately reflects a normal average BMD level — one that actually exists in the population.[21] The result was an average peak bone mass that was much lower than the DXA companies'. This cut the prevalence of osteoporosis, as defined by BMD, by more than half. That is, if researchers had used the manufacturers' reference range in their study, the prevalence of osteoporosis of the hip would have been 49 percent, rather than the 28 percent they found.[22]

The second study, a Canadian government-funded epidemiological study of 10,000 people, set its own population-specific reference standard using a random selection of young women. The results they came up with were equally astonishing. They found the actual prevalence of osteoporosis (as defined by low bone density) to be 16 percent in women and 5 percent in men, as opposed to the official Canadian estimates of 50 percent and 12 percent.[23]

When the researchers of the Canadian study applied the NHANES III criteria for the hip and compared the results to the Canadian criteria, the outcomes were similar. When they were compared with manufacturer's criteria, however, the outcome was vastly different.

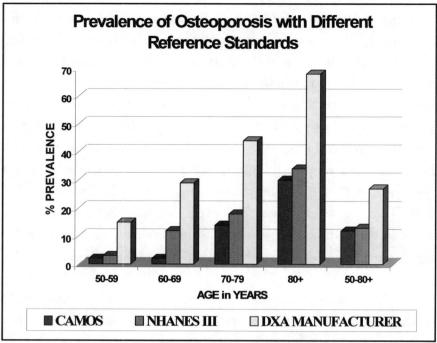

Source: A Tenenhouse. *Osteoporosis International* 2000; 11:897-904. Reproduced with permission.

Estimation of the Prevalence of Low Bone Density in Canadian Women and Men Using a Population-Specific DXA Reference Standard

A study from Turkey shows the prevalence of low BMD fell from 50.3 percent to 14 percent at the spine, and from 60.8 percent to 14.6 percent at the hip, when the manufacturer's standard was compared with a locally produced standard.[24] The authors conclude: "… our data suggest that individual populations should use their own reference range T-scores in DXA in order to avoid misdiagnoses of osteopenia and osteoporosis based on other population's reference range T-scores. Since a low normal BMD is not necessarily indicative of an increased risk of fracture in a given population, this approach might decrease unnecessary patient anxiety and errors concerning treatment."[25]

In a study from the United Kingdom published in 1997, the bone mineral densities of 2,068 women aged 30 to 70 were measured. Fifty-four percent were in the normal range, according to a locally determined standard, but only 25 percent were normal against the manufacturer's standard, leading the researchers to comment: "We observe that manufacturer's reference ranges may not be appropriate for the local population and may lead to an erroneously high diagnosis of osteopenia and osteoporosis, which would lead to unnecessary patient anxiety and perhaps errors regarding treatment."[26]

Another U.K. study reports: "Our findings suggest that patients may be diagnosed as having osteoporosis if one reference range is used but not if another is used, even when the same manufacturer's dual-energy X-ray absorptiometry system is used."[27]

Not surprisingly, some experts are beginning to question the relevance and accuracy of current standards for DXA scanning and the WHO criteria.[28,29,30] Correcting the situation is not simple. They warn that any updates or changes planned to overcome this major problem could make it very difficult to interpret previous readings.[31]

Overall, doctors and general practitioners who recommend bone scanning to their patients are unaware of the controversy, and trustingly make decisions on the basis of the outcome of a DXA scan. The massive discrepancies in the diagnosis of osteoporosis, resulting from inconsistent and inaccurate DXA scanning, raise serious concerns. Many people are being diagnosed with osteoporosis and then treated with prescription medications, when they will never have a fragility fracture.

The Toll on the Patient

The psychological effects of being labeled abnormal or at risk are rarely considered. Such labels cause great distress and anxiety, and are known to "affect the identity and shape the life experience of those who are so labeled."[32] My years as a menopause educator have confirmed the prevailing fear many women have of developing osteoporosis. Their doctors routinely recommend BMD testing as part of the menopause "wellness" package. Once such testing is embarked upon, women are invariably caught in the re-screening loop. An abnormal diagnosis requires repeat testing, which leads to increasing dependency on BMD testing. Hormone replacement therapy or other pharmaceuticals are also likely to be administered over many years to ensure that women retain "normal" levels of bone density.

Susie looked very anxious as she told her story. She had an early menopause, used HRT for only a few months, and then managed the rather difficult transition with exercise and herbal treatments. Ten years later, at age 48, she had been recommended to undergo bone density testing because she was told her early menopause put her at greater risk for osteoporosis. Her bone density measured normal, but she was still worried. Although her bone density was normal, it was at the low end of normal. Because Susie believed she was on the brink of rapid age-related bone loss, she thought the result meant she was still at serious risk for fracture. She could not be reassured. She was convinced by the information from her doctor and the computerized printout from the DXA machine that her bone mass was about to slip from the "normal" range into the "diseased" category.

Accuracy of diagnosis is imperative. Younger perimenopausal women who are identified as having low bone mass in the spine are likely to be encouraged to embark upon treatment. For treatment to be useful, it must be taken long-term. Long-term HRT use is no longer recommended as it exposes women to an increased risk of breast cancer, heart disease, stroke, and other serious complications. Bisphosphonates are not recommended for premenopausal women, and there is no long-term safety data for any age group.

Postmenopausal women had previously reported that the results of bone densitometry testing substantially influenced their decision to begin hormone replacement therapy. A study found that women with moderately low bone loss (osteopenia) were twice as likely to start HRT as women with normal bone mass, and women with very low bone mass (osteoporosis) were more than three times as likely to start.[33]

BMD Testing — Further Limitations

Bone mineral density testing has other limitations as well. The sites most commonly measured are the hip and the spine. But bone density can vary throughout the skeleton. It is hardly conclusive that you have osteoporosis when one part of you, for instance the lower spine, registers low bone density, because the hip may be normal, or vice versa. The NHANES III study found that even different parts of the hip resulted in vastly different measurements. For example, only 10 percent of the population studied had osteoporosis in the whole hip (femur) region, whereas 17 to 20 percent had osteoporosis when each region of the hip was considered separately. In one group of women, 17 percent would have been classified as having osteoporosis in terms of the WHO criteria after having just the neck of the femur scanned, but only 6 percent would have osteoporosis when the entire hip region was scanned.[34]

In the same study, the bone densities of 351 women and 348 men, ranging from 21 to 93 years of age, were measured in 15 body sites — including the spine, hip, wrist, leg, head, pelvis and ribs. Results differed considerably from one site to another, and from men to women. The areas with the lowest BMD were the lumbar spine, the hip, and the wrist. The stage of life when the bone density for a given area was lost was quite different. Bone density in the hip, for example, began to decline very slowly from the age of 20, whereas spinal bone density was stable in women until menopause.[35]

Perspective from Independent Analysts

There are now more than 20 agencies for health technology assessment worldwide, established by governments and organizations responsible for funding health care. These agencies provide rigorous and systematic reviews of the effectiveness of medical interventions to assist them in developing policies that will improve the health of their citizenry. The reports are externally reviewed, and available to the public. The Swedish Council on Technology Assessment in Health Care (SBU) was founded in 1987 while centers at York (NHS Centre for Reviews and Dissemination) and Canada (Canadian Coordinating Office for Health Technology Assessment) were established in the early 1990s. Reports on bone mineral testing and associated treatments have been furnished by 14 such agencies. The British Columbia Office of Health Technology Assessment analyzed findings of 14 major review groups. The office concluded that BMD testing does not result in a reduction of fractures and is therefore not a cost-effective public health strategy.

The following are statements on the usefulness of bone density testing from some of those agencies:

The British Columbia Office of Health Technology Assessment:

Clinical management decisions should not be altered by BMD test results, except in instances where BMD test results may help in the diagnosis of women with symptomatic conditions. In particular, BMD testing should not be used to assist in decisions regarding preventive strategies such as hormone therapy [HRT], nor should it be used to establish a risk assessment of well women. In both of the latter instances, BMD test result will mislabel women more often than not.[36]

The Alberta Heritage Foundation for Medical Research:

There will be substantial numbers of false positives [i.e., diagnoses of osteoporosis] and false negatives [normal when not] when bone density measurement (BDM) is used to assess whether or not an individual is osteoporotic on the basis of the WHO definitions. Many women will be assigned to the wrong category for their risk of fracture.[37]

University of Newcastle Osteoporosis Study Group, Australia:

The measurement of BMD is not a useful screening test for the identification of women at high risk of hip fracture and requiring preventative treatment with estrogens.[38]

Agence Nationale pour le Developpement de l'Evaluation Medicale, France:

Bone mineral density measurement cannot be considered a good screening test (presence of false positives and false negatives decreasing the individual predictive value for fractures).[39]

Swedish Council on Technology Assessment in Health Care:

There is no scientific basis for recommending bone density measurement in mass screening, selective screening, or as an extra component in health checkups of asymptomatic individuals (opportunistic screening).[40]

With reference to the evidence for national screening programs, the independent analysts had this to say:

The International Network of Agencies for Health Technology Assessment:

> When all the scenarios are considered, a BMD screening program aimed at menopausal women might prevent between 1 percent and 7 percent of fractures. Taken together, these estimates of the effectiveness of such a program are not particularly encouraging from a public health perspective and are unlikely to represent good value for the money.[41]

Effective Health Care Bulletin, U.K.:

> It is likely that a bone screening program will lead to the prevention of no more than 5 percent of fractures in elderly women. Given the current evidence, it would be inadvisable to establish a routine population-based bone screening program for menopausal women with the aim of preventing fractures.[42]

The substantial concerns raised by health technology assessment agencies on the effectiveness of bone density measurement and associated treatments warrant close consideration by those concerned with the management of osteoporosis. To date they appear to have had little effect.

A Salutary Tale

The British Columbia Medical Services Commission imposed a moratorium on public funding of bone densitometry (DXA) testing, following the release of a 1996 report by the Office of Health Technology Assessment that called into question the effectiveness of bone density screening. This stopped the growth of BMD technology in publicly-funded facilities in the province for three years. The medical consultant who chaired the British Columbia Ministry of Health at the time was responsible for the moratorium; he was convinced that there was no scientific evidence that BMD testing led to better patient outcomes. In 1999, the medical consultant's contract was not renewed, and he left the ministry. The BMD moratorium ended, and in 1999 the number of publicly funded facilities with BMD-testing capacity doubled. Commercial interests quickly resumed, promoting BMD testing in the province.[43]

Ken Bassett, a member of the BCOHTA group, pays tribute to the medical consultant's decision and its consequences, and warns: "Its outcome reminds us ... about the power and persistence of the private interests whose well-being depends on selling tests and drugs, whatever the evidence might indicate, and of the daunting challenge of attempting to forestall the diffusion of technology that has gained a foothold."[44]

Selective Screening of Well Women

Because of the expense of BMD testing, some countries are encouraging doctors to select well women for screening who are considered to be at higher risk for osteoporosis, rather than all women This is dependent, of course, on the doctor being able to identify the woman at menopause who has a high risk of future fractures, *before* she fractures. Applying risk factors such as a personal and family history of fracture, low body weight, lack of exercise and smoking may help to identify those patients. But as most fractures occur in women long after they have gone through menopause and are due to factors not manifest at that time, there is no evidence to support selective screening.[45]

Other Screening Methods

Bone Remodeling and Bone Markers

Bone is a living organ that is constantly remodeling, replacing, and repairing itself. The adult skeleton is replaced entirely every seven to 10 years. From birth to adolescence and, to a lesser degree, young adulthood, there is massive bone remodeling as we grow taller and the long bones continue to extend. After the adolescent growth period ceases, the bone remodeling process slows, entering the maintenance phase. Then, after menopause, most women appear to have higher levels of bone remodeling once again, although this can vary. In men, the age-related thinning of bones seems to occur about 10 years later than it does in women.

The process of remodeling serves two purposes. First, it keeps bones "young." When you knock your leg or strain to lift a heavy object, the area of bone that bears the impact will begin to repair the micro-damage that has occurred. Second, remodeling makes bone better able to meet the demands placed upon it. This is why a violinist's bow arm, a TV cameraman's holding arm, or a tennis player's racquet arm, all develop bone that is thicker and stronger than the bone of the arm that is less-used.[46]

During the bone remodeling process, certain chemical by-products are produced which can be found in blood and urine. Different chemicals are produced during the bone formation and resorption. These chemicals, called bone markers, have become a relatively new addition to the osteoporosis diagnosis field. By measuring an individual's bone markers, researchers can better gauge if a person's bone resorption is too high or formation is too low, and if treatment is embarked upon, can give some indication of its success after two or three months.

While the accuracy of biochemical markers of bone turnover has improved markedly in the past few years, there is still debate about their application. The general consensus is that measurement of bone turnover markers provides potentially useful information to supplement BMD measurement, but cannot be used to diagnose osteoporosis, evaluate its severity, or select a specific therapy.

Bone Resorption and Formation Markers

Bone is the only organ that has cells designed specifically to destroy it. They are called *osteoclasts*. There are also cells called *osteoblasts*, whose sole purpose is to repair the organ. Healthy bones remodel and repair themselves in much the same way that road maintenance crews repair damaged or weakened roads. Bone is like a well-used highway, which becomes cracked and worn with use and will eventually crumble, unless the cracked and worn patches are removed and replaced. Bone remodeling occurs at sites where damage has occurred as a result of force, as in a knock or fall, or when muscles have been working hard, applying great pressure to bone. Breaking or cracking a bone generates an awe-inspiring sequence of events, which results in complete repair and new, well-formed bone tissue. A certain amount of muscle strain also helps to maintain bone. That is why exercise, particularly weight-bearing, is essential to perpetuate healthy bone remodeling.

The bone maintenance crews are called BMUs (basic multi-cellular units). About one million of these crews are working to remove and replace bone at any one time. When damage occurs in a patch of bone, it is sensed by a network of cells called *osteocytes*, which send signal molecules to alert the BMUs via an extensive "osteo-internet." As in road repair, the first members of the BMU to arrive are the diggers, the osteoclasts, which begin their process of removing damaged bone. This process is known as resorption.

As the osteoclasts dig out the damaged patch, they actually release bone growth-triggering factors that were left there two to five years earlier by cells called osteoblasts, whose purpose it is to rebuild the bone. These factors stimulate new osteoblasts to begin the rebuilding process. The osteoclasts dig tunnels and trenches at the rate of about $1,000^{th}$ of an inch per day. Osteoblasts secrete collagen and laboriously fill in the excavated areas, but take about eight times longer to do so. Gradually, the new bone mineralizes around the new web of collagen and, after about six to nine months, the process is complete.

At certain times of life, there is more bone building than remodeling — as in childhood and youth — so osteoblast cells predominate. Although the full story is not known, it seems that as we age, the BMUs are not as effective at patching and maintaining bone, and we begin to lose more bone than we gain. It is believed that reduced bone density and osteoporosis occur when many factors combine to produce BMUs with deeper-digging osteoclasts and smaller crews of osteoblasts that cannot fill the bigger holes.

Resorption Markers

1. Dpd
As the bone is broken down, a substance called deoxypyridinoline, or Dpd, is excreted in the urine. Dpd is the product of a type of collagen found in bones and is a specific marker of bone breakdown; its levels are unaffected by diet, making it suitable for assessing resorption. Because bones remodel at a higher rate while people sleep, Dpd is measured from a urine sample collected from the first or second urination in the morning. A Dpd score of less than 6.5nM/mM is con-

sidered normal in some labs, based on the levels for healthy men and premenopausal women who are not pregnant. A high Dpd measurement, for adults who are past their bone-growing years, indicates that bone is being lost. Whether the bone-loss rate is cause for alarm is another issue. At present, it is not known whether the Dpd test can predict risk for fracture.

2. Collagen Cross-links (NTX, CTX)
The activity of osteoclasts is measured by breakdown products of collagen. When bone is resorbed, collagen is broken down and fragments that contain the cross-linking molecules are released and excreted in the urine. High levels can indicate high levels of bone resorption.

Formation Markers

1. Bone Alkaline Phosphatase (ALP)
Osteoblastic activity, or bone formation, is associated with osteocalcin, one of the proteins found in relatively high concentrations in bone. Bone alkaline phosphatase (ALP) forms new calcium crystals, and blood levels of this bone enzyme give an indication of new bone formation. However, alkaline phosphatase is formed by many of the body's tissues. Therefore, the routine reporting of ALP levels on liver function tests does not give any information about *bone* alkaline phosphatase. For this, further testing is required.

2. *Propeptide of Type 1 Collagen (PICP)*

Bone is made up of a framework or matrix of interlocking fibers of the protein collagen, which forms the foundation for bone structure, and inorganic components that surround the collagen structure and form the "cement." Collagen is normally flexible and is important in the structure of skin and nails. In bone, however, it is made strong and rigid by tiny crystals of calcium phosphate salts. This relatively new test measures PICP, which is associated with the secretion of collagen. It has been shown to correlate with bone formation.

Diagnostic Methods in Perspective

The connection between bone formation and resorption is poorly understood at present. It is a key puzzle to be solved in the field of bone biology. When a woman is identified with low bone density, it does not automatically mean that she has reduced bone formation and greater bone resorption. Young people can have low bone density, and older people can have higher bone density.[47]

None of these testing methods gives an accurate assessment of bone strength. Because of the great variability in bone turnover, the seasonal variation of bone density, and the day-to-day variation of metabolic processes, these tests cannot accurately assess the risk of a future bone fracture.

Dr. Jane Aubin, a specialist in anatomy and cell biology, and president of the American Society for Bone and Mineral Research, has spent much of her academic life focusing on what causes osteoblasts to form. In a 1998 article, she admitted that science's level of understanding of bone remodeling was at a basic stage. "We are at the tip of the iceberg now," she said. "We don't even know what is in an osteoblast." The article also reported that the basic mechanisms of bone cell change are unknown: "Dr. Antonio Candeliere, one of Dr. Aubin's postdoctoral fellows, added that he has no faith that a DXA scan, measuring bone mass, can tell you much of anything about the structural integrity of bone – whether or not a bone will fracture. 'You've got to do a biopsy to study that.' "[48]

The Doctor's Dilemma

Women accept the advice of their doctors, believing them to be fully informed about the accuracy of methods for diagnosing osteoporosis, and the effectiveness and safety of treatments. Unfortunately, most physicians are not well-informed. Authors of the Alberta Technology Assessment Review comment that the significance and limitations of BMD results seem poorly understood in general practice.[49]

Concerns have also been raised about the interpretation of BMD results. Knowledge of statistics is required, and interpretations can vary from one laboratory and physician to another. A person with osteoporosis can be cared for by her general practitioner, gynecologist, endocrinologist, or a rheumatologist, each with a unique approach to assessing the condition.

> *Women who registered with higher bone density would go on to have 63 percent of all fractures. So, who should be treated?*

The dilemma for physicians is to determine whether low bone density puts their patient at risk for fracture, and therefore whether to recommend treatment. Most doctors are not aware that evidence linking low BMD to fracture is minimal, and that they may do their patient greater harm by prescribing medication. It is hard to argue with the apparent objectivity of a machine. But consider this: The University of Leeds examination of the effectiveness of BMD screening found that of the 20 percent of women with the *lowest* bone density measurements only *28 percent* of those would have gone on to fracture later. Women who registered with higher bone density would have 63 percent of all fractures.[50] So, who should be treated? That is the doctor's dilemma.

✳ 4 ✳

The Myth of Causality

*Myth #3: Age-related bone loss is the cause of deadly
fractures in the elderly.*

Ruth, at the age of 82, underwent DXA bone scan testing at the request of her primary care physician. Her results for the lumbar spine fell in the osteoporosis range and for the hip were in the osteopenia range. She was advised to start taking alendronate (Fosamax). After reading about the side effects of the drug, she wanted a second opinion. She consulted a physician who showed her a study from the New England Journal of Medicine. Citing the article, the doctor informed Ruth that she had no risk factors for osteoporosis other than her age and her low bone density results. Even though her hip bone density was in the range of osteopenia, it was average for women her age. (Her lumbar spine bone density was just below average.) The doctor showed her that even if the drug could improve her bone density from average to the highest third, her risk of a hip fracture would not decrease. She decided not to take the drug.

Like many people, Ruth was concerned about osteoporosis and was afraid of sustaining a fracture, though she had little information about her bone health — other than a measurement of low bone density. This is because physicians and researchers continue to emphasize the single risk factor of low bone density. The concern about osteoporosis, however, is really a concern about fractures. If bone thinned with aging but no one ever fractured, osteoporosis would be an obscure academic subject reserved for the medical texts. Understanding fractures and what causes them is the key issue.

Fractures related to bone fragility tend to occur at sites containing a higher percentage of the porous, honeycomb-like trabecular bone — the predominant bone type in the hip and spine. Other sites that may have fragility fractures are the wrist and the ribs. Fractures of the skull, ankle, and the long bones of the leg are not usually associated with osteoporosis fractures.[1]

Like so many processes, functions and conditions in the human body, the causes of fractures are complex. Blaming fractures on low bone density alone is a gross oversimplification; low bone density is only one of many risk factors. The U.S. National Institutes of Health acknowledges this in a consensus report issued in 2000 titled "Osteoporosis Prevention, Diagnosis, and Therapy." The authors write: "It is important to acknowledge a common misperception that osteoporosis is always the result of bone loss."

Hip Fractures

Hip fractures, among all fragility fractures, result in the greatest suffering to the individual. The evidence is indisputable that hip fractures are severe. The injury has a profound impact on a person's quality of life, as evidenced by findings that 80 percent of women more than 75 years old preferred death to a hip fracture resulting in nursing home placement.[2]

Statistics surrounding hip fractures can be frightening. A 50-year-old woman has a 15 percent chance of fracturing her hip before she dies; a man has a 5 percent to 6 percent risk.[3] Among men and women who live to the age of 90, 32 percent of females and 17 percent of males have experienced a hip fracture.[4] Such statistics, while important, can be misleading because many professionals correlate the increased incidence of hip fracture among the elderly with osteoporosis. In fact, the causes of hip fractures often stem from factors other than age-related bone density loss. Specifically, a person's chance of sustaining a hip fracture can be pinpointed to risk factors associated with falling.

Most hip fractures occur after a fall — even though only 1 percent of all falls in the elderly result in a fracture. About 5 percent of hip fractures appear to be "spontaneous" fractures, in which the patient fractures and then falls. The direction of the fall plays a large role in the outcome. A fall to the side, as opposed to forward or backward, increases the risk of hip fracture by about six times, and is considered a much greater risk than lower bone density.[5]

Dr. Susan Ott, osteoporosis expert, comments: "Other factors include how tall a patient is, how far she falls, how she lands, and maybe the shape of her hip. Also, factors that cannot be measured may be involved, such as how many of the bone cells are alive, how brittle the bone itself is, etc."[6]

The National Institutes of Health, in its 2000 report on osteoporosis, writes:

> Fracture risk has been consistently associated with a history of falls, low physical function such as slow gait speed and decreased quadriceps strength, impaired cognition, impaired vision, and the presence of environmental hazards (e.g., throw rugs).[7]

A British study concludes that the following factors were more accurate than low BMD in predicting hip fracture in the elderly: low body weight, kyphosis, poor circulation in the foot, epilepsy, short-term use of steroids, and poor trunk maneuverability.[8]

Indeed, many of the conditions that increase the likelihood of a person falling (and breaking a hip) can be symptoms of old age: poor eyesight; weakened balance, coordination and strength; and confused mind (often the result of medicinal side effects). The healthier a woman is, the less likely she is to fall and break her hip. Further, the healthier a woman is prior to a fall and hip fracture, the better her chance for recovery.

Popular statistics state that 20 percent to 30 percent of women who break a hip die within a year. Healthy women, however, rarely die from hip fractures. In women who were mobile before a hip or pelvic fracture, it is estimated that as few as 14 percent of their deaths were caused or hastened by the fractures.[9] The mental health of a woman also plays an important role. A British study found that patients with depression, dementia, or delirium appeared to be at increased risk of death after hip fracture. Dr. John Holmes from the University of Leeds conducted the study and concluded that the "findings confirm what is not widely appreciated: that psychiatric illnesses have important effects on physical conditions."[10]

Mechanical Factors

At least half of all of hip fractures after the age of 80 are linked to mechanical factors, not bone fragility. Common cervical fractures, or fractures of the femoral neck, appear to be more related to pelvic structure than osteoporosis — that is, failure of the outer diameter of the femoral neck to expand with age and increased acetabular bone width. Women with trochanteric hip fractures (the wider area of bone at the head of the femur) have a more severe and generalized bone loss due to the greater amount of trabecular bone in that region of the hip.[11] Overall, about half of hip fractures are intertrochanteric, and the others are femoral neck fractures. In older women the proportion of trochanteric fractures increases.

Hip fracture is a function not just of bone density but of the way people fall, of patterns of how weight on the hip is loaded (e.g., squatting), and of such structural features as hip axis length. Many of these aspects vary across cultures. For example, hip fracture risk doubles with each standard deviation increase in hip axis length. Asian adults have shorter hip axes than adult Caucasians; consequently, Asians with the same bone mass as Caucasians have a lower hip fracture risk.[12]

Misleading Statistics

Without wishing to diminish the potentially devastating impact of hip fractures or the seriousness of multiple wedge fractures of the spine, it is important to recognize that fracture statistics, when presented in terms of lifetime risk, are often misleading and needlessly alarming. Bone density loss occurs naturally with age, but not everybody develops thin and brittle bones. Neither are all postmenopausal women at risk for hip fracture. Statistics for hip fractures, when presented in the negative, present a dramatically different picture: 85 percent of women aged 50 with a life expectancy of 80 years will *not* suffer a hip fracture. For those in good health prior to a hip fracture, the injury rarely leads to death.

Risk Factors

It is a myth that low bone density causes fractures in the elderly, especially the most worrisome type of fracture — hip fractures. Understanding that hip fractures result from many risk factors helps a woman overcome the fear induced by a report of low bone density.

Bone health in younger age groups — up to and around menopause — is determined by many factors. For example, a family history of fragility fracture, smoking, inadequate diet, eating disorders, a lack of exercise, side effects of some medications and certain diseases may result in fragile bones.

Risk factors for older people revolve around the increased propensity to fall. An elderly person is more likely to fall under the influence of certain medications. When a person takes multiple prescription medications for a variety of complaints, the effect of drug interaction can compound the problem. Dementia, frailty, and immobility along with low bone density further increase the risk.[13] A study of 9,516 white women over the age of 65 measured the risk factors for hip fracture. The following are listed as the most predictive factors:

- A maternal history of hip fracture
- Having the same body weight as at age 25
- Previous fractures after the age of 50
- Being tall at the age of 25
- Self-rated health being fair or poor
- Previous hyperthyroidism
- Medications — specifically sedatives, antidepressants and long-acting benzodiazepines or anticonvulsant drugs
- Less than four hours a day on feet [14]

Women who had five or more risk factors, including low bone density in the heel, were more likely to have a hip fracture than women who had no more than two risk factors, regardless of bone density.[15] The authors conclude that maintaining body weight, walking for exercise, avoiding medications with harmful side-effects, minimizing caffeine intake, and treating impaired visual function are among steps that may decrease risk.

An Australian study examined risk factors for hip fracture among elderly men and women by looking at alcohol, caffeine, and calcium consumption, and physical activity, smoking, height and weight at different stages of people's lives in order to determine what influence they might have. Investigators found that a history of smoking, being underweight in old age and being overweight at age 20 were linked to an increased risk for hip fracture. Consumption of dairy products, particularly at age 20, was associated with an *increased* risk of hip fracture in old age. The authors comment that this may be because dairy products contain protein. High protein intake can cause breakdown of bone and increase urinary excretion of calcium. Caffeine and alcohol intake were not associated in this study. They conclude that older people can reduce their risk of hip fracture by being reasonably physically active, maintaining a reasonable body weight, and stopping smoking.[16]

The presence of a spine fracture or deformity is considered an important predictor of further fracture. The number of previous vertebral fractures along with low bone density is linked to a greater risk for vertebral fractures, while the severity of previous vertebral fractures alone is the risk factor that predicts non-vertebral (such as hip) fractures.[17]

Treatments

There is no evidence that osteoporosis drug therapies prevent hip fracture in the elderly. Drugs rarely address the major risk factors for hip fracture, such as those factors that increase the likelihood that a person will fall. To prevent fractures, it makes much more sense to consider lifestyle and environmental factors such as:

- Maintaining body weight
- Walking for exercise, remaining active
- Exercising to increase balance and flexibility
- Avoiding long-acting benzodiazepines, corticosteroids, sleeping pills, and other medications, whose side effects either weaken the strength of the bone or impair body function — increasing the chance of a fall.
- Treating impaired vision

- Removing potential tripping hazards in the home
- Consuming a balanced, nutrient-rich diet
- Receiving sunlight exposure or supplemental vitamin D

Hip Pads

In elderly people who are at high risk for fracture, the wearing of a padded undergarment can help prevent such an event. The undergarment incorporates a soft, thin pad over each hip bone and works similarly to the padding in a football player's uniform. The hip pad absorbs the shock of a fall, disperses its impact over a larger area, and reduces the force of a fall on the

> *The elderly group that wore hip pads sustained no fractures, even though they had 5 times as many falls as the control group, which had a 4.3 percent fracture rate.*

vulnerable hip. A recent study found that the frail at-risk group who wore the underwear experienced five times as many falls as the healthier control group — though the at-risk group sustained no fractures. The control group had a 4.3 percent fracture rate.[18]

Despite the effectiveness of the undergarments, they are not widely promoted by doctors. In addition, many elderly people prefer not to wear them because they find them uncomfortable and bulky. A United Kingdom study of 153 residents of residential care homes found that only 3 percent of people would wear them at night and that daytime compliance rates reduced from 47 percent for the first month, to around 30 percent for months five and six.[19] An Iowa study found that with the development of thinner, more efficient pads, this may be less of a problem.[20]

Vertebral Fractures

Vertebral fractures, while not as debilitating as hip fractures, are perhaps equally well-known due to the image of the hunched-over elderly woman with a dowager's hump — a rare condition caused by multiple spinal wedge fractures.

The spine consists of 24 vertebrae, each one cushioned by a flat, cylindrical disk made from cartilage. The larger flat bone at the bottom of the vertebrae is called the sacrum, and the tiny tail bone underneath, the coccyx.

The spine is divided into three sections:

> The cervical spine: the seven vertebrae at the top of the spine that are generally less likely to be affected by osteoporosis.

> The thoracic spine: the 12 vertebrae in the middle of the back that have a pair of ribs attached to each of them. These bones are more prone to abnormality. It is a wedge fracture in the thoracic spine that can form the spinal "hump."

> The lumbar spine: the five vertebrae below the thoracic region. These vertebrae are also susceptible to abnormalities.

Fractures of the vertebrae range from mild to severe. Vertebrae do not usually break apart, so fracture may be a misleading term. Researchers determine vertebral fractures by measuring the height and width of individual vertebra and comparing them to reference ranges. Although criteria vary, if the height of a given vertebra has decreased by more than 3 standard deviations (or 20 percent to 25 percent), it is generally deemed a fracture.[21] Vertebrae tend to compress or become deformed when bone tissue deteriorates with age. Most vertebral deformities occur without any associated pain or major symptoms. Loss of height may occur suddenly or gradually. Most people are unaware that compression has occurred, and so-called fractures are revealed when found incidentally by X-ray. The wedging of vertebrae that causes curvature in the spine can occur normally to some degree with aging and is not necessarily associated with marked bone loss or fragility.[22] Loss of height is most commonly due to thinning of the cartilage discs between the vertebrae and has nothing to do with osteoporosis.

The course of diagnosed spinal osteoporosis is unpredictable, and a low bone density measurement does not predict risk of fracture. DXA scanning technology is not precise enough to identify spinal deformity. This can only be determined with X-ray and careful assessment. Even then, the degree of compression of the vertebra necessary to define an actual vertebral fracture is not standardized. (A height loss of more than 4 centimeters over 10 years has been used by doctors as a way to infer that a vertebral fracture has occurred.) Therefore statistics and research results can vary widely.

In a minority of people, vertebral compression fractures may cause back pain, which generally lasts a few months and can be managed with bed rest and analgesics. The fracture heals, and normal life and activities can be resumed.[23] Spinal back pain may be due to compression fractures, but can also be due to other non-skeletal causes.[24]

In rare, serious cases, the vertebrae become wedge-shaped and an elderly woman may develop a hump in her back after multiple wedge fractures. This is called a dowager's hump and can bring chronic pain and other complications. The image of the hunched-over woman with the dowager's hump has been frequently used in advertising — often with the effect of scaring the women who see such images — but just how common is the condition? According to an Australian study of fragility fractures, the lifetime risk of multiple spinal fractures that cause the dowager's hump is 3 percent.[25] According to the study, the risk of a single fracture, which would not produce the dowager's hump, is 9.6 percent.

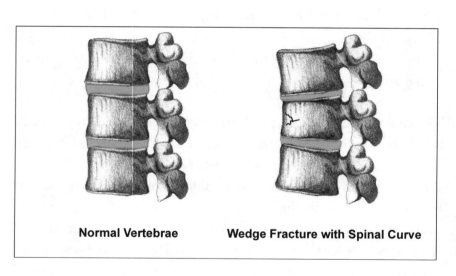

Normal Vertebrae   **Wedge Fracture with Spinal Curve**

Confusing Statistics

Because there is no international standard for defining the degree of compression necessary to establish a vertebral fracture, there is wide variability in rates of fracture.

Dr. Susan Ott comments: "With vertebral fractures the incidence depends on how you measure the vertebra. If you define a fracture as only a small decrease in height, then there will be a lot of them. If you use stricter criteria, then there are not as many. Several good studies have recently been reported showing how much difference it can make."[26]

And even when the same criteria for defining a vertebral fracture is applied, the rates vary widely from one location to the next. In Europe for example, the prevalence of deformities of the vertebrae shows enormous variation from country to country — as much as from 6 to 20 percent.[27] The highest rates are in Scandinavian countries.

To put the incidence of vertebral fracture in perspective, Dr. Bruce Ettinger, osteoporosis expert, writes:

> Clinical vertebral fractures are rare — vertebral deformities based on careful radiographic assessments are much more common. The incidence of the latter [deformities] is about 1 in 200 to 1 in 300 women per year. Clinical fractures are about 1/3 of this rate. The 10 year risk of painful spine fracture for women at age 50 or at age 60 is very low, but the rate increases quite a bit with aging.[28]

Despite such statements, hyperbole and scare tactics proliferate. A search on the Internet produced the following text from a consultant gynecologist:

> Osteoporotic fractures occur in one third of women, principally in the hip (neck of femur), the vertebral bodies and the wrist. Apart from the life-threatening fracture of the hip which occurs in the older age group of women, the collapse fractures of the lumbar and thoracic vertebra produce pain, loss of height, and the deformity of the Dowager's hump. The capacity of the chest is diminished and women have their heart and lungs squashed up into small volume producing greater distress.[29]

Treatments For Vertebral Fractures

Pain medication and rest will assist with the healing process after a vertebral compression fracture. For wedge or compression fractures, the bisphosphonate Fosamax helps reduce the risk of further fractures, but the effectiveness and safety of long-term use is currently unknown.

Two procedures, vertebroplasty and kyphoplasty, have been developed to manage acute vertebral fractures. In the treatments, liquid plastic is injected into the fractured vertebra. The merits of the two relatively new procedures are still being debated. Advocates of the techniques claim frequent acute pain relief. Others express concerns that the long-term effect of one or more reinforced rigid vertebrae could increase the risk of fracture of adjacent vertebrae. There is also a 5 percent risk of "leakage" of the plastic into the spinal cord which could cause serious damage.[30]

Wrist Fractures

Fractures of the wrist are common in women 50 to 70 years old — the age when a woman's balance begins to decline, which can result in a fall. Wrists break when women fall and stretch out their arms to brace themselves. This tends to cause a fracture in the wrist at the end of one of the two bones in the forearm (the radius). This type of fracture is called a Colles' fracture. While other bones in the wrist may fracture, Colle's fractures are the most common. A white woman has a 15 percent chance of fracturing her wrist during her lifetime, according to statistics.

As a woman ages, her reaction time declines; when she falls she is unable to brace herself and is more likely to fall directly onto her hip, rather than on her outstretched arms. Fitness, agility, and speed of gait are also factors. Women who walk faster are more likely to have forward momentum, and if they fall, they land on their wrists.

A Colles' fracture can occur with normal, high, or low bone density of the forearm.[31] Research indicates that factors related to bone geometry rather than bone density are linked to forearm fractures.[32] Wrist fractures, although painful, usually repair successfully. They do not typically have a long-term effect on a woman's quality of life. Neither do they predict subsequent fractures of the hip or spine. They cannot be described as debilitating or devastating, and hardly warrant long-term drug therapy as a preventative measure. To date there is no evidence that current medications will prevent wrist fracture.

Secondary Causes

Osteoporosis is multifactorial. It is a myth that low bone density is the major risk factor for the most serious fracture — the hip fracture, as well as other fractures. In many cases, another underlying medical condition contributes to the loss of bone and bone strength. A diagnosis of severely low bone density may indicate that some other condition, disease, or disorder is behind it and may increase a person's likelihood of fracture. These are known as *secondary* causes.

In pre- and perimenopausal women, more than 50 percent of osteoporosis (low bone density) is associated with secondary causes, the most common of which are: glucocorticoid drugs, steroids that are prescribed for conditions ranging from asthma to arthritis; thyroid hormone excess; antiepileptic therapy; and low estrogen levels, often the result of a surgical removal of the ovaries.[33]

In cases where young people fracture easily and have low bone mass, there is commonly a secondary cause. For instance, many young people who take prednisone and other glucocorticoids are at risk. Such medications have been known to weaken bone. The U.S. National Institutes of Health have raised concerns about this issue and have advocated development of glucocorticoids that avoid deteriorating the skeleton.[34]

In postmenopausal women, the prevalence of secondary conditions is thought to be lower. In reality, however, it is not known, as doctors often fail to test for secondary causes after postmenopausal status has been determined. Diagnosis is commonly made on the basis of a bone density test alone. Consequently, statistics concerning secondary causes in this demographic of women are hard to come by. However, in one study of postmenopausal women, researchers identified several factors that contributed to the loss of bone, including: hypercalciuria, (the excretion of abnormally large amounts of calcium in the urine), hyperparathyroidism (the over production of parathyroid hormone by the parathyroid glands), and malabsorption (poor absorption of nutrients via the digestive system). These women were found to have low bone mineral density.[35]

Osteoporosis in men is usually related to secondary causes such as alcoholism, hypogonadism, and glucocorticoid treatments for asthma, rheumatoid arthritis, inflammations, and other ailments.[36] Studies estimate that 30 to 60 percent of osteoporosis in men is associated with secondary causes. Researchers have started to examine whether low levels of male hormones contribute to bone loss. Testosterone in particular, like estrogen, is implicated in bone loss. Testosterone increases muscle mass, which indirectly results in higher bone density. Testosterone is also converted to estrogen, which in turn influences bone resorption.

A study of 355 men more than 60 years old revealed several secondary causes which contributed to lower bone density, including: previous fractures, gastrectomy, peptic ulcer disease, rheumatoid arthritis, glucocorticoid use, hypertension, previous hyperthyroidism, height loss since age 20, chronic lung disease, and smoking.[37]

Medical Conditions

A number of medical conditions are associated with lowered bone density and increased risk of fracture:

- hormone disorders such as hyperparathyroidism, hyperthyroidism, hypothyroidism
- gastrointestinal diseases such as celiac disease
- cystic fibrosis
- blood disorders
- genetic disorders
- connective tissue disease such as rheumatoid arthritis
- nutritional deficiencies
- a variety of other common serious chronic systemic disorders, such as congestive heart failure, end-stage renal disease, and alcoholism.

Drugs

A major factor often overlooked in people who are considered "normal," yet fracture easily, is the issue of prescription drugs. The list of drugs which cause bone loss includes: alcohol, aluminum, anti-seizure medications, cyclosporine A, exchange resins, lithium, luteinizing hormone-releasing hormone agonists, medroxyprogesterone acetate (Depo-Provera), methotrexate, neuroleptics used to treat schizophrenia, steroids such as glucocorticoids, and thyroid hormone (excess).[38]

Glucocorticoids (Corticosteroids)

Glucocorticoid use is the most common form of drug-related osteoporosis. The steroid is widely used for long-term disorders such as rheumatoid arthritis and other connective tissue diseases, asthma, psoriasis, Crohn's disease, lung disease, inflammatory bowel diseases, severe allergic reactions and inflammations, obstructive pulmonary disease, and in organ transplants. Corticosteroid treatment causes bone loss by a variety of complex mechanisms. Within the first year after starting corticosteroid therapy, patients lose on average 14 percent of their bone mineral content. Up to *50 percent* of patients using the drug may fracture, especially postmenopausal women.[39]

Patients treated with 10 milligrams of the corticosteroid prednisone for just 20 weeks experienced an 8 percent loss of BMD in the spine. High dose treatment (greater than the average daily dose of 7.5 milligrams prednisone) has been shown to increase a patient's risk of developing vertebral fractures more than four-fold and to double the risk of experiencing a hip fracture. Investigators found that even lower daily doses of corticosteroids (between 2.5 milligrams and 7.5 milligrams) increased the risk of vertebral fractures by 2.5 times. In addition, these lower-dose levels increased a patient's risk of developing a hip fracture by more than 75 percent.[40]

Some experts suggest that any patient who receives orally administered glucocorticoids (such as prednisone or cortisol) in a dose of 5 milligrams or more for longer than two months is at high risk for excessive bone loss. People who have undergone organ transplant are at high risk for osteoporosis due to a variety of factors, including pre-transplant organ failure and use of glucocorticoids after transplantation. The long-term effects on bone of intermittent use of systemic steroids or the chronic use of inhaled steroids, as are often used in asthma, are not known.[41]

Depo-Provera (Medroxyprogesterone Acetate)

Depo-Provera is a contraceptive injection usually given every three months and also commonly used to treat premenstrual syndrome (PMS), pelvic pain syndrome, endometriosis, and advanced breast cancer in premenopausal women. It has been found to reduce bone density in young women by up to 4.1 percent per year, although bone density increases again once the treatment is stopped. Concerns have been raised about women using the drug around menopause, when bone density is naturally decreasing and is unlikely to recover in the same way as it does in a younger person when the treatment stops.[42]

Heparin

Continued use in high doses of the blood-thinning drug heparin is associated with reduced bone density and osteoporosis-related fracture. Warfarin, another anticoagulant, has not been reported to have these effects.[43]

Antacids

Taking large doses of antacids can cause severe bone pain, rickets (osteomalacia), and fractures. Stopping the treatment will rapidly improve symptoms.

Thyroid Hormone (L-Thyroxine) Replacement Therapy.

Several studies have shown that long-term thyroxine therapy given to women with hypothyroidism may decrease bone density, particularly in postmenopausal women.[44]

Vitamin D Deficiency

Vitamin D, sometimes called a hormone and sometimes a nutrient, helps to control the formation of bone tissue. It increases the amount of calcium and phosphorus the body absorbs from the small intestine and thus helps regulate the growth, hardening, and repair of the bones. (See Chapter 10 on Creating Strong Bones for more information on vitamin D.)

Thyroid Conditions

The thyroid gland, located in the neck below the Adam's apple area, regulates metabolism. It secretes hormones to help cells convert oxygen and calories into energy. A woman faces as high as a 1-in-5 chance of developing thyroid problems during her lifetime. That risk increases with age and for those with a family history of thyroid problems. Women may suffer from hyper- (too much) or hypo- (too little) thyroid hormones. Hyperthyroidism, an excess of circulating thyroid hormone, is a well-known risk factor for osteoporosis. Too much thyroid hormone increases metabolism to the point where more bone is destroyed than is created. Hyperthyroidism affects about 2 percent of women and 0.2 percent of men. Treatment for hyperthyroidism often involves surgery or ablation of the gland with radioactive iodine. Both procedures can result in hypothyroidism. There is evidence that women taking thyroid replacement medication for hypothyroidism may be at increased risk for excess bone loss, suggesting that careful regulation of thyroid replacement is important.[45]

Hyperparathyroidism

Though the names are similar, the thyroid and parathyroid glands are separate glands, each producing distinct hormones with specific functions. The parathyroid glands are four pea-sized glands located on the thyroid gland in the neck. The parathyroid glands secrete parathyroid hormone (PTH), a substance that helps maintain the correct balance of calcium and phosphorous in the body. PTH regulates release of the calcium from bone, absorption of calcium in the intestine, and excretion of calcium in the urine. When the amount of calcium in the blood falls too low, the parathyroid glands secrete just enough PTH to restore the balance.

If the glands secrete too much hormone, as in hyperparathyroidism, the balance is disrupted and blood calcium rises. This condition of excessive calcium in the blood, called hypercalcemia, or in the urine (hypercalciuria), indicates that something may be wrong with the parathyroid glands. The excess PTH triggers the release of too much calcium into the bloodstream. As a result, the bones may lose calcium, and too much calcium may be absorbed from food. The levels of calcium may increase in the urine causing kidney stones. PTH also acts to lower blood phosphorous levels by increasing excretion of phosphorus in the urine.

Menstrual Irregularities in Young Women

Failure to achieve peak bone mass, bone loss, and increased fracture rates have been evident in young women who have abnormal patterns of menstruation. Low levels of female hormones in a young woman brought about by delayed start of menstruation, very few menstrual periods, or an absence of menstrual periods are relatively common in adolescent girls and young women. These can occur as a result of strenuous athletic training, emotional stress, and low body weight.

Eating Disorders

Anorexia nervosa and bulimia are conditions which particularly affect young people, and can have devastating consequences. They are usually involve an abnormal fear of obesity, a distorted body image, and abnormal eating patterns such as obsessive fasting, self-induced vomiting, or the use of laxatives. The effects of these disorders range from mild weight loss to delayed sexual development, heart problems, depression, osteoporosis (low bone density), and even death.

Research has indicated that the condition might result in bone mass loss in up to 90 percent of anorexic women. Tests of 130 young women with anorexia showed that 38 percent of them had osteoporosis as defined by bone mineral density. The researchers from Massachusetts General Hospital indicated that 92 percent of the women showed bone mass loss at the hip, the spine and the extremities. The research indicated that supplementary female hormones (HRT) did not reduce the risk of bone mass loss in these women.[46] The investigators conclude that in these women body weight, not estrogen deficiency, is a significant predictor of bone mineral density, and stress that anorexic women should be counseled about the adverse effects of low weight on the skeleton.[47]

In a statement from Massachusetts General Hospital, Boston, Dr. Anne Klibanski, one of the principal researchers says: "Some of these young women are experiencing bone loss comparable to that of women many decades older, despite estrogen therapy. Given this severity and the prevalence of bone loss, the importance of screening all women with anorexia for osteoporosis cannot be over-emphasized."

Celiac Disease

Celiac disease is a genetic disorder of the small bowel or the duodenum. The digestive tract is damaged by gluten proteins from wheat and other grains and is unable to effectively absorb nutrients including essential minerals for healthy bones. Celiac disease can account for a spectrum of illnesses ranging from relatively mild digestive symptoms to more serious conditions including osteoporosis, anemia, and diabetes. It is often undiagnosed because of its many mild and varied symptoms. Celiac disease can be simply and effectively reversed with the adoption of a gluten-free diet.

Evidence from the largest study ever conducted on the prevalence of celiac disease in the United States reveals that approximately one in every 133 Americans has the condition. The study maintains that only one out of 4,700 Americans has been diagnosed, meaning that 97 *percent* of cases go undetected.[48] Because many physicians don't consider celiac disease in determining a cause for osteoporosis, it is reasonable to conclude that a correctable cause of low bone density is being overlooked. In an Italian study, 86 newly diagnosed celiac disease patients, 66 percent of whom were found to have osteoporosis (low BMD) or osteopenia, adopted a gluten-free diet and then had their bones scanned again after one year. The gluten-free diet led to significant improvement in bone mineral density, even in postmenopausal women.[49]

Other Causes

Cystic fibrosis and inflammatory bowel disease are examples of conditions associated with malabsorption and resultant low bone density in some individuals. The osteoporosis of cystic fibrosis is also related

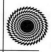

to the frequent need for corticosteroids as well as to other undefined factors.

The Myth of Causality

Low bone density is one of many risk factors for fracture, and often a minor one. The focus on low bone density has led to the myth that age-related bone loss is the major cause of fracture and that it must be treated. Often eliminating other risk factors and secondary causes of bone loss can do more to prevent fracture than attempting to increase bone density via medication. The excessive attention to low bone density has shifted the focus from modifiable risk factors to drug therapies. These therapies, discussed in the following chapters, come with their own set of concerns and problems.

Section II: Treatment Myths

✳ 5 ✳

Overview of Drug Treatments

My sister Barbara, at age 56, is one of millions of women who have been diagnosed with osteoporosis. Her bone density is very low, and she has been strongly encouraged to take the bisphosphonate drug Fosamax long term. She has no vertebral fractures and hasn't fractured since she was 7 years old. She has no other risk factors for osteoporosis. She writes: "When I was first diagnosed with osteopenia prior to menopause, I felt in a state of shock. The DXA scans showed I was well below the average, and I was told it was likely my bone density would reduce even further after menopause. My doctor wanted to prescribe HRT, but I didn't want to take it."

Barbara's doctor believed that HRT would slow down her bone density loss as she went through menopause and reduce her risk for fracture later. She had reservations about using HRT because she had heard conflicting reports about its safety. We now know she was right to trust her instincts. New evidence for serious risks associated with HRT has meant that women taking it long term to prevent osteoporosis are being advised to stop.

Hormone Replacement Therapy

Forty years ago, the Western world thought that medicine had discovered the Holy Grail in the form of supplemental estrogen — a hormone treatment claiming to halt the aging process, alleviate menopausal symptoms and prevent postmenopausal health risks.

The production of the hormones estrogen and progesterone by the ovaries naturally decreases with the onset of menopause, and after menopause the body achieves a stable, but different, balance of hormones. With the availability of prescription female hormones however, a whole medical paradigm was developed around the concept of the "estrogen-deficient woman," based on the questionable theory that once a woman is postmenopausal she requires regular doses of hormones to bring her back to "normal."

HRT was initially heralded as a health-promoting tonic that would prevent a variety of serious conditions while simultaneously keeping users young. Doctors the world over embraced estrogen replacement (and later combined estrogen with progesterone) while massive marketing campaigns successfully appealed to women's vanity and desire for "eternal youth." For many health-conscious women, HRT became the accepted way to manage the ups and downs of the menopause transition — the hot flashes, sweats, sleep disturbances, mood swings, and vaginal dryness — while simultaneously "preventing" heart disease and osteoporosis.

The Risks of HRT Use

Breast Cancer
Breast tissue is known to be sensitive to reproductive hormones. For this reason there has long been concern about breast cancer risk among women who take HRT. The WHI trial found a 26 percent increase of invasive breast cancer after three years (8 more cases annually among 10,000 women using HRT). It has been noted that if investigators had considered only the women who stayed on the trial and not included the absentee 42 percent who dropped out, there was actually a *50 percent increase* in breast cancer — almost double the risk stated in the published results.[24] Women are offered the reassurance that HRT is not believed to increase deaths from breast cancer among women who are regularly screened so that breast cancers are diagnosed early. However, HRT alters breast tissue density and is associated with a higher rate of wrong diagnoses — negative and positive. An Australian study found that the sensitivity of mammography at detecting cancer is significantly lower in HRT users, especially in women aged 50 to 69 years old.[25] It is also worth noting that modest alcohol consumption and HRT use is associated with an increased risk of breast cancer.[26]

Ovarian Cancer
A U.S. study that examined 44,241 women for approximately 20 years found that women using estrogen-only therapy had a 60 percent greater risk of developing ovarian cancer. The risk increased with the length of use. Another study of 46,260 postmenopausal women that looked at the number of deaths from ovarian cancer in those taking estrogen alone found that more than 10 years use was associated with an increased risk of ovarian cancer that persisted up to 29 years after cessation of use.[27] The risk of ovarian cancer was approximately doubled in women who had used estrogen for 10 or more years, but was not evident in less than 10 years of use. The impact of HRT (combined estrogen and progesterone) on ovarian cancer risk is unknown.

Endometrial Cancer
For users of estrogen-only replacement, there is a three- to five-fold increased risk for endometrial cancer (cancer of the lining of the womb). Risks increase with duration of HRT use. This risk is avoided by adding progesterone to the HRT regimen in women with an intact uterus.[28] Women who have not had a hysterectomy should not use estrogen alone.

Although justification for use came from trials that were poorly designed or lacked controls, the medical community had become convinced that HRT would prevent age-related heart disease and osteoporosis. Early studies claimed to show a reduced risk for heart disease, the number one killer of women in the United States. And when HRT was found to slow bone density loss through the menopause transition, normal age-related bone loss was identified as a major cause of osteoporosis in older women. Consequently, many

Risks of HRT (cont.)

Heart Disease
Coronary heart disease is the leading cause of death among women. In the WHI study, healthy women who took combined HRT had a higher rate of fatal and nonfatal heart attacks within the first year of use. The study found that heart disease increased by 29 percent in HRT users — or, to seven more heart attacks in 10,000 HRT users every year.

Previously, a large four-year, placebo-controlled trial had shown no benefit overall to women with established risk factors for heart disease. It did however show a significantly higher incidence of fatal heart attack in the first year of use, along with increased deep venous thrombosis (DVT), pulmonary embolism, and gallbladder disease in the HRT group.[29] HRT is no longer recommended for the treatment of heart disease.

Stroke
The WHI trial found that strokes increased in women using HRT by 41 percent after two years, resulting in eight more strokes among 10,000 users annually. New evidence from the trial casts more bad light on combined HRT. Stroke risk was found to be elevated during all five years of the study, and was increased by 53 percent in the first year.[30] Twenty years of follow-up in the Nurses' Health Study had previously shown that higher daily estrogen doses of 0.625 milligrams or more along with progesterone may increase the risk of stroke by up to 45 percent.[31]

Blood Clots (Venous Thromboembolism)
Five out of six studies looking at the effects of HRT on clotting have reported that the risk is highest in the first year of use. Most commonly these blood clots occur in the legs and are called a deep venous thrombosis, or DVT. The danger with a DVT is that the clot can break loose and travel to the lungs. In that case, it can interfere with breathing and cause death. The results from these studies reflect the findings from the WHI trial, which reported a 100 percent increase in clotting of the legs and lungs in the first year. This is equal to 18 more cases of clotting annually in 10,000 women using HRT.[32]

Other Risks
There is evidence from the on-going Nurses Health Study that HRT causes an increased risk of gallstone formation among current and long-term HRT users. The risk is also higher among women who have stopped using HRT.[33] Women who use HRT also have a two-fold increased risk of developing lupus erythematosus.[34] Because of the threefold-increased blood clotting risk, it is recommended that HRT be withheld for 90 days after any surgery.[35] Recent analysis of data from the Women's Health Initiative indicated that women using estrogen alone or combined HRT had a greater risk of asthma than women not taking hormones.[36]

women were advised to undergo a long-term HRT regimen to replace the "missing" bone-protective hormones, and to protect their hearts.

The promise that a single pill could prevent age-related chronic diseases was so compelling that many millions of healthy women proceeded to take HRT long term for diseases they didn't actually have and may never have developed. By 2001, hormone replacement therapy was the No. 1 prescription drug *in the world*.[1] By 2002, 38 percent of postmenopausal United States women (some 16 million) were using hormone replacement therapy, making it the most frequently prescribed medication in the United States, accounting for more than $1 billion in sales.[2] But that was about to change.

There had always been something of a disconnection between the evidence for HRT and the zeal with which doctors prescribed it. Research showed that HRT relieved hot flashes and, in a local application, treated vaginal dryness in postmenopausal women. However, no large clinical trials had proven that the therapy prevented heart disease and fractures, and there was no credible evidence that HRT improved memory, mental clarity, incontinence, depressive symptoms, skin age, libido, or overall well-being.[3] Perhaps most importantly, the long-term effects of the treatment were unknown.

The combined estrogen and progestin branch of The Women's Health Initiative trial (WHI), one of the largest clinical trials of its kind ever undertaken in the United States, was halted prematurely after 5 years in July 2002, when interim results indicated that HRT significantly increased the risk of serious disease. The study of 16,608 healthy women aged 50 to 79 found the HRT group had a 41 percent increase in strokes, 29 percent increase in heart attacks, 100 percent increase in the rates of venous thromboembolism (blood clots), 22 percent increase in cardiovascular disease, and 26 percent increase in invasive breast cancer when compared to women taking a placebo. The trial also reported a 24 percent reduction in fractures and a 37 percent decreased risk of bowel cancer.[3,4]

On releasing the findings, Dr. Jacques Rossouw, the acting director of the Women's Health Initiative said: "The WHI results tell us that during one year, among 10,000 postmenopausal women with a uterus who are taking estrogen plus progestin, 8 more will have invasive breast cancer, 7 more will have a heart attack, 8 more will have a stroke, and 18 more will have blood clots, including 8 with blood clots in the lungs, than will a similar group of 10,000 women not taking these hormones. This is a relatively small annual increase in risk for an individual woman. However, even small individual increases over time, and on a population-wide basis, add up to tens of thousands of these serious adverse health events."[5]

The trial sponsors, the National Institutes of Health, concluded that the risks of long-term use outweighed the benefits, and an editorial in the Journal of the American Medical Association concluded: "The WHI provides an important health answer for generations of healthy postmenopausal women to come — do not use estrogen/progestin to prevent chronic disease [i.e., osteoporosis and heart disease]."[6]

Adriane Fugh-Berman, M.D. and Cynthia Pearson ask the obvious question in their article, "The Over-Selling of Hormone Replacement Therapy," published in the October 2002 issue of Pharmacotherapy. "Why did the medical and research community ever believe that hormone replacement therapy (HRT) prevented or treated disease? Not a single controlled trial ever showed that HRT prevented cardiovascular disease, stroke, Alzheimer's disease, or wrinkles, nor that it was an effective treatment for depression or incontinence."[7]

What about fractures? It is true that HRT slows bone density loss in most women who use it. But reducing bone loss and preventing fractures are two very different goals in managing osteoporosis. Until the results from the WHI trial in 2002, there was no evidence from randomized controlled trials that HRT prevented fracture. In fact, a large clinical trial had found that, after four years, HRT did not show any anti-fracture benefit, and in 2001, the FDA had withdrawn its approval of HRT as a treatment for osteoporosis.[8,9]

Although the WHI trial found that the women using HRT had fewer fractures overall, it has not changed the FDA recommendation. The U.S. Preventative Services Task Force analysis of the WHI trial report concluded that the reductions for hip and vertebral fracture "did not achieve statistical significance in adjusted analyses." They state that the differences in fracture rates between placebo and HRT groups were so small that it depends on the criteria that are applied whether the results are significant. The task force also advises that because of the concerns surrounding long-term safety, HRT should not be used for the prevention of osteoporosis.[10] The FDA, which has done its own analysis of the WHI results, has asked that labels on both estrogen and estrogen-progesterone replacement therapy be revised to carry a "black box" warning noting the increased risks for heart disease, heart attacks, strokes, and breast cancer. This applies to all brands and types of hormones.

Postmenopausal Women Are Not Hormone Deficient

It is important to understand that women are not "hormone deficient" after menopause. The endocrine system of the body is exquisitely orchestrated, and a number of hormones interact constantly to maintain it. The ovaries go on producing lesser amounts of estrogen, and androgens produced by the adrenal glands are converted into a weak form of estrogen by fat cells in the body. A study published in the New England Journal of Medicine indicated that the majority of women over 65 produce enough estrogen naturally to give them bone protection.[11]

Whether altered or lowered levels of hormones cause fragility fractures is questionable. When the hormone levels of postmenopausal Mayan women of Central America were measured, they were found to have estrogen levels no higher than those of white American women — even lower in some cases. They live for an average of 30 years after menopause, and they don't lose height, don't develop a dowager's hump, and don't get fractures. Bone density tests showed that they lost bone density at the same rate as U.S. women.[12]

If osteoporosis-related fractures are due to estrogen deficiency, it would be reasonable to expect that women with the disease have lower levels of estrogen than women without the disorder. This is not the case. Studies have found that estrogen levels are similar in postmenopausal women with and without osteoporosis.[13]

All women go through menopause, but not all women are at risk for fracture. African-American women, for example, have a two-fold lower risk of fracture, and in countries like Ghana, Guinea, and the Democratic Republic of the Congo, osteoporosis is extremely rare. Asian women have lower rates of fracture, and Hispanic women have approximately half as many fractures as Caucasian women.

Women can expect to feel wonderfully well after menopause. Many women say they have never felt so well, optimistic, energetic, fit, and strong. Gone are the swings in energy and mood, the hot flashes, and the complications of menstruating and menopause. In their place is a sense of wellness and enthusiasm for life. My sister maintains that the joys of being a postmenopausal woman are one of those well-kept secrets — something that she and her contemporaries share, while modern medicine tends to view it as a stage of life requiring regular monitoring for disease.

The Case for Current Osteoporosis Treatments

Barbara went for another scan after menopause. "Some years later another DXA scan had shown further lowering of my bone density particularly in the lower spine, and in addition to suggesting HRT, my physician also recommended the bisphospho-nate Fosamax as a treatment option. He said there was 'a clear case for one or the other.' Feeling bolder after having refused to take HRT, I had arrived at the appoint-ment with a folder of notes and a clipboard with my sheet of questions. I proceeded to take notes as he answered my questions, pausing and checking with him to make sure I had understood what he meant. At one stage, he leaned over his desk, took my paper, and wrote the name of the drug we were discussing on my paper. 'FOSAMAX.' At the time, I felt his action intrusive and patronizing. It was a gesture I have not for-gotten. I was being told by an expert that I had a serious condition that required what sounded like drastic long-term treatment, when I felt perfectly healthy. In addition, I knew by then that there were major questions around the effects and the value of this treatment."

Following the results of the WHI trial, for the millions of women who were taking HRT, and for those diagnosed with low bone den-sity, the question has become "What do I do now?" Many are being encouraged to begin treatments such as Fosamax and Evista, but need to know if the drugs are safe and effective. Despite what the adver-tisements say, the answers are not straightforward. In fact, when examining the current treatments for osteoporosis, a paradox emerges: although they may influence bone density, they do not ben-efit the majority of people taking them. It is even possible they may exacerbate a patient's condition.

Drug treatments prescribed for osteoporosis continue to focus on bone density — an aspect of bone health that reveals little about the micro-structure and strength of bones. Treatments aim to slow bone density loss and in some cases increase bone density, yet no conclusive evidence exists that any of the treatments will prevent fractures in an individual with low bone density. Neither is there evidence that these treatments will rebuild fragile bone. Drugs that can increase bone density are not able to reverse the loss of bone strength that occurs in the type of osteoporosis where the trabecular struts are severed; no bone agent has been shown to rebuild severed connections.[14] Thus, a treatment that significantly increases bone density will not necessarily reduce fracture rates, alleviate pain, or prevent disability.

> *Treatment that significantly increases bone density will not necessarily reduce fracture rates, pain, or disability.*

More than 10 years ago studies were done to measure the effect of sodium fluoride on bone. Fluoride was well-known for its ability to increase bone mineral density, which explained why the compound was added to tooth-paste and why many cities fluori-dated their drinking water. Many osteoporosis experts felt that long-term studies of its effect on fracture rates were not necessary. However, the studies found that fluoride did not reduce the incidence of fractures — even though it caused huge increases in spinal bone mineral density. In fact, fracture rates were *higher* among people taking fluoride than those taking a placebo. Apparently, fluoride helped create new bone of poor quality.[15] Fluoride is no longer considered a treatment option.

Evidence proving the effectiveness of osteoporosis treatments is far from conclusive. To date, research indicates a limited reduction in the risk for vertebral fractures in older women with osteoporosis who have *also* had a previous vertebral fracture. But scant evidence exists for any treatment that can reduce hip fractures.

Why, then, do some treatments claim to significantly increase bone density or significantly reduce fractures? It is helpful to understand that in medicine the word "significant" carries a specific meaning: that *the measured change is unlikely to have occurred by chance.*

> *Scant evidence exists for any treatment that can reduce hip fractures.*

When a result is "statistically significant," it does not mean that the change or benefit was large, or that the studied population received any noticeable benefit. It just means that the drug has brought about a change that has been demonstrated to be true beyond a reasonable doubt. Thus, if a treatment has been shown to significantly increase bone density, it doesn't mean it will make a difference to the life of the individual who takes it.

Claims that a certain drug will "prevent" fracture really mean that the drug reduces a person's *risk* for fracture by a certain percentage. An advertisement for Fosamax, the bisphosphonate drug alendronate, claims that in clinical tests women with low bone density who took Fosamax experienced 44 percent fewer vertebral fractures compared to women receiving a placebo. That sounds impressive, but in reality, the benefit was very small. How can that be? In the large Fosamax trial, called the Fracture Intervention Trial, after three years, 2.1 percent (43 women) taking Fosamax suffered a vertebral fracture, compared with 3.8 percent (78 women) who took the placebo. This was a difference of 35 fractures among 4,134 women. The reduction stated in the advertisement was 44 percent less, but it was 44 percent of the already small 3.8 percent fracture rate.[16] The actual reduction in fractures is only 1.7 percent.

When these results were released, many experts concluded that the Fosamax trial showed no benefit at all. The minimal reduction in fractures — many of which were vertebral fractures detected on X-ray and

not necessarily the type of fracture that causes pain or symptoms —
did not provide sufficient evidence to treat.[17]

What is Your Chance of Preventing Fracture?

One way to examine the effectiveness of a treatment is to consider
the numbers needed to treat, or NNT. This medical term refers to
the number of patients who must be treated to prevent, in this case,
one fracture in one person over a defined number of years. The
NNTs tell an interesting story.

Here's an example. Fosamax is also claimed to reduce hip fractures
by 50 percent. In a study of 2,027 postmenopausal women with
osteoporosis and previous fracture, after three years there were 22
hip fractures in the women who took placebo (2.2 percent), and 11
in the Fosamax group (1.1 percent). The actual reduction was 1 percent, not 50 percent. Based on these statistics *90 women* would need
to be treated for three years to prevent one hip fracture. The remaining 89 would receive no benefit.[18]

If a woman has low bone density (osteopenia), but no previous fractures, her risk for fracture is low. Any treatment is going to margin-
ally reduce an already low risk. It is estimated that around 60 such
women would need to be treated for three years to prevent one vertebral fracture in one of them.[19] When a woman has very low bone
density and has had previous fragility fractures (osteoporosis), her
risk for fracture is much higher. Even so, it is estimated that 15
women would need to undergo treatment for three years to prevent
one vertebral fracture in one of them.[20] It is estimated that *hundreds* of
women in their 50s with low bone density or osteopenia would need
to be treated more than three years to prevent one hip fracture in one

woman. That means that hundreds would be taking a drug, exposing themselves to side effects, and receiving no benefit.[21]

Osteoporosis expert Dr. Ego Seeman of the University of Melbourne, Australia, poses the question: "Should we expose huge numbers of these women [age 50 and with low bone density] to a drug, its costs, inconveniences, side-effects, when most will not sustain a fracture had no treatment been given? That is, most who take the drug will be exposed to the risk of side effects and costs and receive no benefit ... This is the nature of preventive medicine; we have to treat large numbers to avert events in few. This is why the drugs we use must be safe — because most exposed do not benefit, and even a small number of adverse events can tip the balance of net benefit to net harm."[22]

Are Current Treatments Safe?

Many medications carry side effects — at times, quite serious ones. Who hasn't heard the expression, "The cure is worse than the disease"? Researchers try to uncover a drug's side effects prior to submitting it for approval to the FDA. However, unanticipated side effects can surface long after a drug has been approved, as illustrated by the recently confirmed risks of hormone replacement therapy.

Treatments for osteoporosis are relatively new, and few long-term studies have been conducted. Consequently, the debate continues over long-term side effects for many treatments. For example, the first-line treatments for osteoporosis currently are the bisphosphonates alendronate and risedronate — the most potent of the antiresorptive drugs, because they slow down the normal bone remodeling process. Bone remodeling removes any micro-damage in the bone and is essential for maintaining healthy bone. There is now evidence that bisphosphonates prevent the routine removal of micro-damage, which may be causing an accumulation of microfractures. There are concerns that long-term use may reduce bone strength and actually increase fractures. Dr. Seeman warns: "Whether the drugs we use in osteoporosis reduce fractures long-term, i.e., 5 to 10 years of therapy, remains unresolved. Therefore, the justification for long-term treatment on the basis of scientific data is unclear. We still need to answer the following question: Do drugs that suppress bone remodeling reduce or increase the risk of fracture in the long term?"[23] The research that answers this question has yet to be done; most studies last a few years at most.

Making an Informed Choice

Ten million people in the United States have been diagnosed with osteoporosis, and health officials estimate that at least 33 million more men and women have undiagnosed low bone density and are at increased risk for osteoporosis. Health officials are urging doctors to identify at-risk patients and proceed with "bone sparing" treatments.

Making the decision to embark on osteoporosis treatment is complex and difficult. The information that follows on current therapy options needs to be viewed in the light of the previous points made in Chapters 1 – 4. Namely, low bone density is not a disease requiring treatment, and a genuine diagnosis of established osteoporosis (bone fracture) is often linked to other factors that should be addressed before considering treatment. Many of these factors involve lifestyle choices that can help create healthy bone and are discussed in Chapter 10. Ultimately, the decision to undergo treatment must involve a careful weighing of the risk for fracture against the risk of embarking on a treatment with unknown long-term side effects that cannot guarantee prevention of fracture.

* 6 *

The Myth of Safety

Myth #4: Osteoporosis can be safely treated and prevented with drugs.

In the wake of the results of the Women's Health Initiative trial, many women previously taking HRT are seeking information about other forms of osteoporosis prevention and treatment. A shift in physician prescribing patterns is occurring, and there is a need for credible information about available therapies.

Bisphosphonates

Bisphosphonates are non-hormonal drugs that are now replacing HRT as the osteoporosis treatment of choice. Alendronate (or Fosamax) and risedronate (or Actonel) are the two bisphosphonates that have been approved by the FDA for the treatment of osteoporosis. They are considered appropriate for use by both women and men, and are also indicated for treatment of Paget's disease, hypercalcemia, skeletal metastatic disease, and other bone diseases.

Other bisphosphonates include etidronate, ibandronate, pamidronate, and zolendronate. More are being developed. Bisphosphonates are synthetic compounds that bind to bone mineral crystals and inhibit bone resorption. They are known to be effective in slowing bone loss and can increase bone density in the short term. A patient using bisphosphonates gets "one shot" to increase bone density; continued use of the drug appears to only maintain bone density.

Although there is evidence for a reduction in vertebral fractures in older women with previous vertebral fracture (in the first three years of use), there are currently no long-term placebo-controlled studies completed that indicate what the benefits or risks beyond five years might be. This lack of long-term safety data and the way in which bisphosphonates suppress bone turnover are causing some experts to advocate caution in their use.

Bisphosphonates can have unpleasant side effects, and administration can be difficult. It is necessary to accept a strict regimen to prevent potentially serious stomach problems and to maximize absorption. The drugs must be taken on an empty stomach. Food must be avoided for up to two hours. It is necessary to remain upright for at least 30 minutes because of the risk of irritating or even making holes in the wall of the esophagus. Recently, a once-weekly, rather than a daily, dose of both alendronate and risedronate has been approved by the FDA. Some bisphosphonates are administered by injection.

How Do They Work?

Bisphosphonates inhibit the action of osteoclast cells, slowing bone resorption. In other words, the drugs disrupt the mechanism that allows osteoclasts to remove old, weakened bone, so that osteoblast cells can build new bone. But osteoblasts *require* the activity of osteoclasts and the resorption of old bone to trigger their activity. In the absence of osteoclasts, osteoblasts are eventually immobilized. This explains the increase in bone density that occurs in the first year or so of use, but also explains the subsequent plateau effect. New bone can only be built after old bone is removed. When bone removal ceases, the bone remodeling process largely ceases.

Evidence suggests that this suppression of bone remodeling may reduce bone toughness and increase microfractures, which could in turn increase bone fragility.[1] Although it is not known whether this effect reduces bone strength, there are concerns that long-term use of bisphosphonates will produce an older skeleton with more crystallized bone that will have less tensile strength in places like the hip. Osteoporosis authority Dr. Ego Seeman cautions that "over time, this process may produce a thinned and brittle structure that may be prone to structural failure."[2] There are fears that fracture rates may begin to increase again with longer use. Osteoporosis expert Dr. Susan Ott advises: "In adult women with osteoporosis the bisphosphonates are effective for 4.5 years, but maybe not longer than that, more data is really needed. Up to 7 years no serious side effects have been seen, but there might be more vertebral fractures during years 6 to 7."[3]

Bisphosphonates, like alendronate, deposit in the bone for more than 10 years, and accumulate with use. Stopping treatment does not remove them from the body, and their influence would continue for better or worse. At the same time, short-term use of bisphosphonates is not recommended because the bone quickly returns to its original state. Dr. Susan Ott cautions: "I do not think it is wise to give alendronate for longer than 4.5 years. I would have to see definite proof of safety and benefit to the bones (in terms of fractures) before I would give it longer than that."[4]

Bisphosphonates and Young People

To date, pharmaceutical options for young people diagnosed with osteoporosis are virtually nonexistent, although bisphosphonates are being studied on young populations in some countries. Because bisphosphonates suppress normal bone remodeling, there is potential for these drugs to harm the young, growing skeleton. In addition, there is concerning evidence that bisphosphonates given to young women or women of childbearing age may actually cause abnormalities in the skeleton of the unborn child. As bisphosphonates, such as alendronate, can remain in the body for more than 10 years after being taken, some experts are advising great caution in prescribing the drug to any younger or premenopausal women.[5] A diagnosis of low bone density in a young person is not necessarily a cause for concern unless it occurs in the presence of other risk factors such as fragility fracture, abnormal thyroid and parathyroid function, etc. Little is known about osteoporosis in young people, and attention to good nutrition, lifestyle, and exercise is of primary importance.

My daughter Camille's situation remained of greatest concern for me in all my research. By the time she was 20, she was urged by the specialist to begin treatment to increase her very low bone density. It was explained to us that the available therapies were still experimental and it was probable, but not certain, that they would be effective. We were assured, however, that they were safe. She was offered a bisphosphonate called pamidronate that would be administered twice yearly by injection. She was eager to begin treatment, but I was not at all certain or convinced that this was the

right thing to do. Despite warnings that time was running out for her, I convinced her to let me research the therapy. After a long period of research, I found information that deeply disturbed me. Bisphosphonates like pamidronate should not be given to younger women. Because these drugs suppress the natural remodeling process of bone, they could cause Camille's bone to age, become brittle, and fracture more easily. They are drugs that stay many years in the body once taken, so stopping them would not reverse the effect. Most alarming for a young woman of childbearing years, there is evidence that the drug can harm the developing fetus by causing abnormalities in the skeleton as it is forming.

Alendronate (Fosamax)

Alendronate appears to increase bone mass in the short term, but evidence for effectiveness in preventing fracture is limited. The four-year, placebo-controlled Fracture Intervention Trial (FIT) enrolled 6,000 women of average age 68 years with low bone density at the hip. There were two arms to the study: 2,000 women who already had vertebral compression fractures and 4,000 women who had not.[6,7] Bone density increased in 90 percent of women taking the medication, whether or not they already had a fracture.

> *It is estimated that 60 women with low BMD would need to be treated for 3 years in order to prevent one fracture discernible by X-ray.*

In older women with osteoporosis and previous vertebral fracture, there was a 7 percent reduction in further vertebral fractures in those using alendronate. This means that 22 women would need to take the drug for three years to prevent one vertebral fracture discernible by X-ray. In women with low bone density but no previous fracture, there was little evidence for benefit. It is estimated that 60 older women would need to be treated for three years in order to prevent one fracture discernible by X-ray. Alendronate appeared to *increase* the risk of wrist fractures in this trial, and there is little evidence for a reduction in hip fractures. Most of the clinical trials of Alendronate have not enrolled women older than 80 years, the group most at risk for hip fracture.

> *If bone density were the main risk factor for osteoporosis, it would be expected that after 4.5 years of increased bone density, there would be a noticeable reduction in fractures.*

Expert commentary on this study from Dr. R. Heaney cautions that the results are minimal: "The anti-fracture benefit of bisphosphonates in women with low bone mass but without prevalent fractures must be judged to be small."[8] In the same commentary, the point is made that, although bone density increased in the patients taking alendronate or Fosamax, it did not make a significant difference to fracture incidence. If bone density were the main risk factor for osteoporosis, it would be expected that after 4.5 years of increased bone density, there would be a noticeable reduction in fractures.

Fosamax's Side Effects

Two studies found that nearly 1 in 3 women using alendronate daily to treat osteoporosis complained of severe digestive reactions, including irritation, inflammation, or ulceration of the esophagus.[9] Side effects from daily use have caused many users to stop taking the medication within a matter of months. Signs of ulceration include throat pain, difficulty swallowing, chest pain, and heartburn. In addition, these studies showed that 56 percent of women fail to comply with the strict dosing guidelines. Recently once-weekly doses have been approved by the FDA. They have been found to be as effective as a daily dose, with fewer upper gastrointestinal side effects. However, the two-year studies of weekly therapy have not been large enough to determine the effect on fracture reduction.

Alendronate may also cause problems when combined with other drugs. In one study, researchers found that 10 milligrams per day of alendronate plus 500 milligrams of naproxen (a non-steroidal, anti-inflammatory drug) twice daily, produced ulcers in 38 percent of the volunteers and significant side effects in 69 percent. The researchers conclude that alendronate and naproxen act synergistically in inducing stomach ulcers.[10] Naproxen is one class of drugs often given to treat arthritis and other pain syndromes. It is not uncommon for older women to be prescribed these types of medications — sometimes for the pain of vertebral fractures.

Alendronate has also been linked to hypocalcemia (abnormally low blood calcium concentration), increased parathyroid hormone, and skin rash.

Risedronate (Actonel)

Two separate placebo-controlled studies have found that risedronate increases bone mineral density and reduces the incidence of vertebral fractures in women who have had previous vertebral fractures. The results are similar to those found with alendronate.[11,12] More recently, a study of postmenopausal women with low bone density but no previous fractures found that three years of risedronate reduced the risk of first vertebral fracture. The researchers advise that 15 such women would need to be treated for three years to prevent one such fracture.[13]

> *If 100 women took risedronate for 3 years, it would save just over one hip fracture.*

However, a study measuring the effect of risedronate on hip fracture in 5,445 elderly women found small benefit only. After three years of use, women less than 80 years old with osteoporosis had a 1.9 percent incidence of hip fracture compared with 3.2 percent of the placebo group.[14] In other words, if 100 women took the drug for three years, it would save just over one hip fracture. Women less than 80 years old with low bone density and previous fracture had a better result. Their risk of hip fracture was reduced from 5.7 percent to 2.3 percent. However, in women more than 80 years old, the age when they are at much higher risk for a hip fracture, risedronate did not significantly decrease hip fracture risk.

The same concerns about long-term use of alendronate apply to risedronate. That is, there is no long-term safety information, and no evidence that risedronate will prevent fracture in the long run.

Risedronate's Side Effects

Risedronate has the same administration requirements as alendronate. To avoid injury to the esophagus, it must be taken on an empty stomach with a full glass of water while in an upright position. The patient must not lie down for at least 30 minutes after taking the medication. The most commonly reported side effects with risedronate are back pain, nausea, headache, peripheral edema, diarrhea, and abdominal pain.

Selective Estrogen Receptor Modulators (SERMS)

Raloxifene

Raloxifene or Evista, is one of a drug class known as selective estrogen receptor modulators or SERMS. SERMS are anti-estrogenic — that is, they work differently from estrogen in that they don't appear to cause an increase of cancer cells in the breast, but still have an anti-resorptive effect on bone.

As often happens in medicine, a drug prescribed for a certain purpose will show risks and benefits in unexpected ways. Tamoxifen is also a SERM and is prescribed for women who have had breast cancer. In the late 1980s, researchers noted that women taking tamoxifen had increased bone density.

Since then, Raloxifene has been developed as treatment specifically for osteoporosis. It has been approved by the FDA for prevention of postmenopausal bone loss. It is believed that it may produce some of the beneficial effects of HRT, without the

> *There is no evidence that Raloxifene will prevent hip fracture, the most worrisome type of fracture.*

adverse effects. But at this time, treatment with raloxifene has not been shown to decrease the risk of either breast cancer or cardiovascular disease in early postmenopausal women.

The Multiple Outcomes of Raloxifene Evaluation (MORE) study involving 7,705 postmenopausal women is the largest osteoporosis trial ever conducted. The participants averaged 70 years of age and had all been diagnosed with osteoporosis. Raloxifene increased bone density by 3 percent and reduced vertebral fractures by about 40 percent after three to four years. In other words, 22 women with osteoporosis would need to be treated for four years to prevent one of them having a vertebral fracture. In the group with low bone density and previous vertebral fracture, the number needed to treat is 12.[15] There is no evidence that Raloxifene will prevent hip fracture.

Raloxifene's Side Effects

Raloxifene can increase menopausal symptoms of hot flashes and leg cramps by 50 percent, and also poses a threefold-increased risk for venous thrombosis or clotting — similar to that found with HRT. Unlike tamoxifen, raloxifene does not appear to stimulate the lining of the uterus, and is therefore less likely to be associated with an increased risk of cancer of the uterus.

Other FDA-Approved Treatments

Parathyroid Hormone (PTH)

In November 2002, teriparatide therapy (Forteo), which is a synthetic form of parathyroid hormone, was approved by the FDA as the newest treatment for osteoporosis. It will be offered to people with severe osteoporosis or those who have already fractured. Currently treatment lasts for two years. There are potentially serious risks associated with use, and there is no long-term safety data at this time.

The action of parathyroid hormone treatment (PTH) is different from other osteoporosis drugs that are classified as "anti-resorptive" treatments that affect bone loss. PTH treatment stimulates bone formation, and for reasons that are not fully understood, daily injected low-doses of PTH appear to stimulate bone formation more than resorption, and may even rebuild trabecular bone.

PTH treatment appears to significantly reduce vertebral and non-vertebral fractures. In a recent study of women with severe osteoporosis, those given the drug experienced a 65 percent reduction in spinal or vertebral fractures while other fractures declined 53 percent.[16] Patients are required to give themselves daily injections using needles, much like those used by diabetics.

The new drug also comes with a "black box" warning on the packaging. When rats were injected with high doses of the medication, they developed a rare bone cancer. But the FDA says the tumors were not seen in any of the 2,000 men and women who used the drug for up to a year and a half. For this reason, treatment is currently not recommended for more than two years. There is also concern that the increase in bone turnover and associated increase in bone porosity with PTH use may offset some of the apparent positive effects on bone strength.[17]

In trials, Forteo was associated with a slight increase in dizziness, leg cramps, headache, and nausea.

Calcitonin

Calcitonin is a natural hormone found in our bodies. It is made by the thyroid gland and controls the activity of osteoclasts, the cells that reabsorb bone. Calcitonin is also found in certain fish, including salmon, and has been extracted for use as a drug to treat the bone disease known as Paget's Disease, and also osteoporosis. Salmon calcitonin was first approved for the treatment of osteoporosis in 1984 in the United States. It appears to have few risks associated with use.

Although previously administered by injection, a nasal spray form of calcitonin has been approved for the treatment of osteoporosis in women who are five years postmenopause. A placebo-controlled trial of 1,255 postmenopausal women with low bone density and one or more previous vertebral fractures found that calcitonin treatment slowed bone density loss and reduced new vertebral fractures over a five-year period. There is no evidence of hip fracture prevention.[18] Calcitonin has been found to have analgesic qualities in the management of severe pain due to vertebral crush fractures.[19]

When osteoporosis has occurred as a result of treatment from corticosteroids, calcitonin may be an effective treatment. A recent study showed that calcitonin appears to preserve bone mass in the first year of glucocorticoid therapy at the lumbar spine by about 3 percent compared to placebo, but not at the femoral neck (hip).[20]

The most common side effects are nasal dryness and irritation, back and joint pain, and headache. It is advised that the drug should be administered with calcium and vitamin D.

Calcitriol

Vitamin D is necessary for the proper absorption and use of calcium in the body. It is accessed through ultraviolet light, and a few food sources such as milk. Some studies suggest that vitamin D deficiency is very common, particularly in populations with limited sun exposure.

A metabolite or derivative of vitamin D, calcitriol increases the intestinal absorption of calcium, and has been advocated for the treatment of osteoporosis, as it has been considered to stimulate bone formation.

There is limited evidence that calcitriol treatment may reduce vertebral fractures. At this time, it is recommended that treatment with both vitamin D and calcitriol be restricted to supervised use by patients with limited sunlight exposure and patients with above normal vitamin D requirements.

There is the potential for kidney damage with long-term use, and it can cause high levels of calcium in the urine.

Experimental Treatments

Fluoride

There is considerable controversy about the effects of fluoride on bone strength and fracture risk. It one of the few treatments known to stimulate osteoblast activity and actually increase bone density — an apparently desirable outcome. But increased bone density does not necessarily mean stronger bone. Experience with fluoride has shown that past a certain point, bone may in fact become more brittle and fracture more easily.

> *Increased bone density does not necessarily mean stronger bone.*

In her Web site, Osteoporosis and Bone Physiology, Dr. Susan Ott writes:

> In a large well-designed randomized, blinded clinical trial, women who used fluoride for four years had increased fracture rates compared to placebo controls. The bone density of the spine increased by 32 percent, but the hip did not show increased density and the rate of hip fractures was nearly three times as high in the fluoride group. At this time fluoride cannot be recommended for clinical use. Because it is one of the few medications that can enhance osteoblast activity, it thus deserves further research.[21]

There is some evidence that fluoridated water is linked to an increased risk of hip fracture, suggesting that even exposure to low levels of fluoride may put elderly people at greater risk.[22] A 1995 study of elderly women in 75 parishes in southwestern France found that the risk of hip fracture was 86 percent greater in those areas with water fluoride concentrations above 0.11 parts per million (ppm).[23] Optimal concentrations of fluoride in U.S. drinking water are considered to be between 0.7 and 1.2 milligrams per liter (0.11 milligrams per liter (mg/L) is the same as 0.11 parts per million).[24]

Strontium Ranelate

Strontium ranelate is a new drug that appears to reduce the incidence of vertebral fractures in postmenopausal women with low bone density. The precise architectural changes of bone resulting from strontium ranelate treatment have not yet been reported, but like PTH, strontium ranelate appears to decrease bone resorption and stimulate bone formation at the same time. Researchers conducted a recent three-year trial of 1,649 women, most of whom had a previous fracture. They found that after one year of treatment, 44 women experienced a new vertebral fracture in the treatment group, compared with 85 in the placebo group. After three years, 139 had a new vertebral fracture in the treatment group compared with 222 in the placebo group.[25] There did not appear to be any significant adverse effects. It is not clear whether it is useful in the treatment of hip fractures. Patients also received calcium and vitamin D supplements daily. Strontium ranelate does not have FDA approval at the time of this writing.

Estren

The synthetic compound estren appears to increase bone density and strength in female and male mice. Researchers report that the drug works similarly to hormone replacement therapy, but doesn't appear to have HRT's risks for cancer and heart disease. It is still in the early stages of testing and is part of a new class of compounds called ANGELS (Activators of Non-Genomic Estrogen-Like Signaling). Further animal research may result in estren becoming another osteoporosis treatment.

Growth Hormone

Controversial human growth hormone treatment may also be added to the list of treatment options for osteoporosis. Research indicates that growth hormone increases bone remodeling and may help during late postmenopause, when there is decreased bone turnover. Currently, however, results from studies are mixed, and its role in maintaining normal levels of bone density is uncertain. In some cases, bone density has increased modestly. Using growth hormone to prevent physiological bone loss that occurs with aging seems possible, but has to be debated more fully.[26]

Progesterone

In recent years, natural progesterone has become popular among women, some doctors, and practitioners of natural medicine. It is used for the treatment of menopause symptoms and has been recommended for the prevention of osteoporosis. Natural progesterone is synthesized in a laboratory from the wild yam or from soy. It is what is known as a "nature identical" hormone, because its molecular structure is identical to the hormone progesterone produced by the ovaries. In this way, it differs from the progestin used in HRT and hormonal contraceptives, which usually have a slightly altered molecular structure.

There has been some evidence that progesterone enhances the formation of new bone.[27] Progestins (progestagens) used in HRT and contraceptives have been reported to prevent or reverse bone loss in certain clinical situations.[28] But in young women taking injectable medroxyprogesterone acetate (Depo-Provera) for contraception, their bone density was found to be 7 percent lower than young women not using the drug.[29]

The popularity of progesterone is based largely on the work and the writings of Dr. John Lee, who reported that applying progesterone to the skin in the form of a cream was almost always successful in increasing bone mineral density in postmenopausal women. In his study, 100 women used the cream during a three-year period. Sixty-three of the women had bone density tests that indicated an average bone density increase of 15.4 percent over the three-year period, compared with an expected loss of 4.5 percent. Most of the women had previously fractured, but no new fractures were reported during the three-year study.[30] This study was conducted as an observational study — that is, there was no control group. For this reason, the results of observational studies are not viewed by the research community as definitive.

In addition to the progesterone, the women in the study were encouraged to consume green, leafy vegetables; to avoid cigarettes and carbonated beverages; to supplement with calcium, vitamin D, and vitamin C; and to participate in a regular exercise program. Some of the women were also taking estrogen. Because each of these additional recommendations may have a positive influence on bone density, it is difficult to say whether it was the progesterone or the combination of the strategies that had the effect.

In a more recent, randomized controlled trial in the United States, 102 healthy postmenopausal women used progesterone cream and calcium and vitamin supplements. During the one-year study, there was no significant difference in bone density between the progesterone and the control groups.[31]

It appears that transdermal natural progesterone, either by itself or in combination with calcium and a multivitamin, has little or no effect on bone mineral density. In the absence of long-term safety data, nature identical hormones must be considered to carry the same risks as conventional HRT.

> *It appears that transdermal natural progesterone, either by itself or in combination with calcium and a multivitamin, has little or no effect on bone mineral density.*

DHEA

DHEA and DHEAS are steroid hormones secreted by the adrenal cortex. Levels peak between the ages of 20 to 30 years. Levels decline steadily thereafter, and at 70 years are found to be less than 20 percent of the peak values. Several studies have shown that supplementation with DHEA strengthens the immune system, heightens brain activity, and improves overall well-being. An increase in levels of estrogen in postmenopausal women after supplementation with DHEA has been noted as a possible link to increasing bone density. At this time, there are no studies to confirm the effect. As always, in the absence of long-term studies, concerns are raised about the safety of taking supplemental doses of the hormone.[32]

Ipriflavone

Many women are using isoflavones made from soy and other plant sources for menopause, and as a protection against bone loss. Ipriflavone is a synthetic "isoflavone" that until recently showed promise as an osteoporosis treatment. A recent randomized controlled trial of 474 postmenopausal women is considered the definitive trial on ipriflavone. Designed to investigate its effectiveness and safety, the trial found little to recommend it.[33] No difference in bone density was seen between the two groups, and in an adverse outcome, some of the women taking ipriflavone had lower levels of certain white blood cells (lymphocytes that are an important part of the immune system) than those taking the placebo.

Summary

While newspaper, magazine, television, and radio advertisements claim effectiveness for the many treatments offered for osteoporosis prevention and treatment, most have little data to support their use, at this time. The worrying lack of evidence from long-term studies should dissuade most women from considering these types of treatments. A diagnosis of low bone density alone is not sufficient reason, given that most fracture risk is not related to bone density. Much of the risk can be minimized without having to resort to drug therapy. Many simple, positive steps can be taken to create bone health that will not only benefit a woman's skeleton, but will also benefit her overall health and well-being.

�֍ 7 ✣

The Myth of the Magic Bullet

Myth #5: The myth that high calcium intake alone prevents osteoporosis, whether from dairy or supplements.

When it comes to creating bone health through nutrition, one piece of advice seems to drown out all others: "Calcium, particularly from dairy products, builds strong bones." That message is driven home to children and, increasingly, adults — thanks largely to the California Department of Food and Agriculture, which formed the California Milk Processor Board in 1993 to make milk more competitive and increase consumption. Its advertising campaign, franchised nationally since 1995, features celebrities, athletes and movie stars on billboards and in magazines with the famous milk moustache, under the heading, "Got Milk?" The real question, of course, is, "Got Healthy Bones?" — a question of immense concern for everyone wanting to avoid osteoporosis.

Much of the discourse and research concerning nutrition as it relates to bone health, including osteoporosis, has focused on calcium — and with good reason: A mature male skeleton contains more than 1,400 grams of calcium (about 3.1 pounds); a mature female skeleton contains more than 1,200 grams of calcium (about 2.6 pounds). In fact, 99 percent of the body's calcium is found in the bones and teeth. The remaining 1 percent of calcium circulates in the blood and has many significant functions. Calcium helps regulate the heartbeat, nervous system, muscle control, enzyme systems, and hormone secretions. Calcium helps cells to cohere and blood to coagulate. If the body lacks enough circulating calcium for these functions, it leaches it from the bones. Even a slight drop in blood calcium levels stimulates the release of calcium from the bones and its absorption from the intestine, at the same time decreasing its loss into the urine. The process is reversed through the actions of vitamin D, calcitonin, estrogen, and other hormones. In this way bone mineral content is continuously being replenished.

Getting the recommended daily allowance of calcium at all ages is important, preferably from dietary sources. Over the years, however, calcium intake alone has been equated with bone health — another example of the "magic bullet" approach in which a complex condition is solved by a miracle drug or a single nutritional ingredient. In this milieu, many women think that diet has little to do with osteoporosis beyond measuring the calcium levels of foods. Bone nutritional requirements are much more complex than that, and preventing osteoporosis involves far more than drinking milk on a regular basis. Consider, for example:

- Most women with osteoporosis get plenty of calcium.[1]

- Calcium supplementation alone is not proven to build bone.[2]

- Countries with the highest rates of osteoporosis are the biggest consumers of dairy products.[3]

In reality, bones are complex, dynamic, and alive, and have a wide range of nutritional needs. It is puzzling that the diverse nutritional needs of bone are often ignored, and that those at risk for osteoporosis are regularly advised to supplement with calcium alone. Two of the most important issues that often get overlooked are the body's ability to effectively absorb calcium and how much excess calcium will be excreted from the body — factors which can vary hugely from individual to individual.

An Exquisite Balancing Act

To sustain life, the level of calcium in the blood must be kept within a very narrow range. This is achieved by an exquisitely orchestrated mechanism involving parathyroid hormone and vitamin D, which maintains skeletal calcium and blood calcium in a state of equilibrium.

The body maintains a balance after adjusting for diet, intestinal absorption, excretion, and hormonal functions, as well as growth, physical activity, and disease. For example, research indicates that people excrete between 150 and 250 milligrams of calcium per day — an amount that can fluctuate, depending on factors such as how much protein and sodium a person consumes.

Vitamin D controls the amount of calcium in the bones. A person who ingests low levels of calcium will have increased levels of circulating calcitriol to improve calcium absorption, whereas a person who receives high levels of calcium will have depressed levels of calcitriol and the calcium will be inefficiently used. People with high-calcium diets excrete more calcium than people with low-calcium intakes, which perhaps explains why osteoporosis is not rampant in countries where people receive low amounts of dietary calcium.[4]

Children, Calcium, and Healthy Bones

> *The beneficial effect of physical activity may dominate as a determinant of bone mass and bone density early in life.*

Many nutrients and mechanisms are involved in the building of peak bone mass in a young person, and even when there is a low calcium intake, a normal peak bone mass can be achieved. Studies of children with low calcium and vitamin D intake in developed and developing countries show that children still achieve a normal peak bone mass despite an apparently deficient diet. The author of a review of the evidence for this phenomenon comments, "It is nearly impossible to explain the robust skeletal mass obtained by so many youngsters who have known nutritional inadequacies of calcium and vitamin D but who are otherwise healthy and active. Nature must somehow be providing well for skeletal growth despite limited intake of the critical nutrient calcium during periods of bone development." He concludes: "The beneficial effect of physical activity may dominate as a determinant of bone mass and bone density early in life."[5]

Increasing Calcium is Not the Answer

Because the amount of calcium in the blood is so carefully regulated, increasing calcium does not necessarily mean that the body will build more bone. Researchers in Madison, Wisconsin, measured the diets and the bone densities of 300 premenopausal women aged 20 to 39, and found that high-calcium diets did not result in higher bone density.[6] In fact, too much calcium (more than 2,000 milligrams daily over a long time) can be detrimental. Taken to excess, calcium can cause kidney stones and gallstones. Studies of countries with highest rates of hip fracture reveal that they also have the highest dietary intake of calcium — mainly from dairy products.[7] This is probably because a high intake of animal protein increases urinary excretion of calcium. It may also be linked to dietary sodium (salt) intake.

Seriously low calcium intake may lead to deficient bone formation, but this is not borne out by observations of cultures with low calcium intake. It is generally agreed that calcium intake within the normal dietary range appears to be adequate for bone health. High dietary calcium intake has not been shown to lead to stronger bones.[8] The recommended daily allowance (RDA) for calcium is 1,200 milligrams.

Whether calcium supplementation actually affects bone density is an ongoing debate. Studies have shown both positive and negative results. It would appear that taking calcium, whether as a supplement or via dairy products, seems to have little bone-density-increasing effect unless a person's diet is grossly calcium deficient. Most studies have shown that calcium supplementation has little effect on the bone density of the spine, and no effect on the bone density of the hip, the two places where most serious breaks occur.[9] The calcium intake in the Netherlands is high and so is the incidence of osteoporosis.[10] In fact, a low dietary calcium intake and low BMD have been linked to fewer fractures in Asia and Africa, as well as populations in the United States and Europe.[11]

A study of women in Pittsburgh, Pennsylvania, confirmed that taking a calcium supplement is only part of the story — having the body absorb it is another. Researchers found that the intake of fat and fiber significantly influences calcium absorption. Surprisingly, women with a higher fat intake and a lower intake of fiber absorbed more calcium. Only certain types of fiber, like wheat bran, seem to reduce calcium absorption. Other forms, such as the fiber found in green, leafy vegetables, including kale, broccoli, and bok choy, did not appear to be detrimental. Women with high blood levels of vitamin D also showed increased absorption, while women with high alcohol intake showed decreased absorption.

Calcium intake alone does not protect against osteoporosis. Nor does low calcium intake predict fracture risk. A 1992 review of fracture rates in many countries showed that populations with the lowest calcium intakes had far fewer fractures than those with higher intakes.[12] For example, black South Africans had a very low average calcium intake — only 196 milligrams — yet their fracture incidence was far below that of either black or white Americans.

Consider these facts:

- Osteoporosis incidence (as defined by fracture) is highest in those countries where the most (dairy) calcium is consumed: the United States, Australia, New Zealand, Switzerland, the United Kingdom, and Northern Europe.[13]

- In Gambia, the average bone mineral density and calcium intake is very low, yet, so is the incidence of osteoporosis (fracture).[14] This finding may be explained by the fact that animal protein intake is lower — therefore the calcium requirement is lower.

Minimizing Calcium Loss

For the vast majority of people, creating healthy bones can be attained by limiting calcium loss. To date, however, researchers have focused on how much calcium gets ingested in relation to the amount of bone formed. Understanding how and why the body loses bone is essential. Two case studies illustrate how calcium consumption alone fails to account for bone health.

Inuit peoples have a normal to very high intake of dietary calcium — between 500 and 2,500 milligrams per day — and one of the world's highest intakes of protein — between 250 and 400 grams per day. They also have one of the very highest rates of osteoporosis in the world (as defined by bone mineral density).[15]

African Bantu women, on the other hand, take in only 350 milligrams of calcium per day, compared to the recommended daily amount of 1,200 milligrams. Yet, Bantu women never have calcium deficiency, seldom break a bone, and rarely lose a tooth. They consume much less calcium and much less protein than Western populations, and yet are essentially free of osteoporosis (fractures).[16]

How can this be? The answer can be found by examining the diets of the two cultures. The Inuit subsist on a meat-based diet consisting of caribou, sea mammals, fish, and birds. The Bantu consume a vegetarian-based diet. Research shows that meat-based diets increase the acidity in the blood and urine, as indicated by a lower pH, a measurement indicating the degree of acidity and alkalinity. People who eat meat have an average urine pH of between 4.5 and 5.5, whereas people who do not eat meat have a pH of between 5.5 and 6.5. To buffer the higher acidity and regain equilibrium, the body leaches calcium from the bones. Studies in the United States that compare women who eat meat-based diets with those who eat vegetarian-based diets reach the same conclusion. Vegetarian women experience half the bone loss of women who eat meat.[17]

Maximizing Calcium Absorption

For calcium to help bone growth, the body must be able to absorb it efficiently. Calcium absorption varies enormously from person to person. Clinical trials of postmenopausal women have found that calcium absorption can vary by as much as 61 percent, and that 40 percent of women in calcium balance trials could not absorb enough calcium to stay in balance even with an intake of 800 milligrams per day.[18] This means that those who could not stay in balance were losing calcium from their bones. Researchers suggest that the women could not absorb proper levels of calcium due to their high intake of dietary salt or protein, among other reasons. The study highlights the importance of considering the multitude of other factors when treating osteoporosis. Poor intestinal absorption of calcium may also occur with celiac disease, or gluten intolerance, which remains undetected in many people.

The food one eats plays a major role in calcium absorption. Most importantly, the amount of protein and sodium (salt) we eat will affect how much calcium is lost in the urine. Protein from meat, milk, and eggs contain relatively high concentrations of sulfur amino acids. As previously discussed, the consumption of this form of protein causes the urine to become more acidic, and can lead to the increased loss of calcium in the urine. Therefore, people who have low protein or sodium diets may require lower calcium intakes than those on high protein diets. A 1994 report in the American Journal of Clinical Nutrition showed that when animal proteins were eliminated from the diet, calcium losses were cut in half.[19]

The role of phosphorus in osteoporosis is unclear, though researchers believe that a dietary ratio of roughly an equal amount of calcium to phosphorus is necessary to maintain normal calcium levels. Because meats contain large amounts of phosphorus, excessive consumption of meat may therefore affect calcium balance. Phosphates in carbonated drinks can have a similar effect, and there is evidence that teenagers and children who consume carbonated drinks high in phosphoric acid have restricted calcium absorption. Researchers at the Harvard Medical School have found that cola drink consumption increases fracture rates in young girls in the United States.[20]

Smoking also causes calcium to be lost from the bone and could result in a higher rate of fracture. Researchers studying the bone densities of identical twins found that long-term smokers had a 44 percent greater risk of fracture than their nonsmoking twins.[21]

Studies also indicate that people who reduce their salt sodium intake to 1–2 grams per day cut their calcium requirement by an average of 169 milligrams per day. For every gram of dietary salt consumed, approximately 26 milligrams of calcium is lost in the urine. And for each gram of

> *Moving to a low-salt, low-protein, vegetarian diet can reduce calcium requirements by over 370 milligrams per day.*

animal protein consumed, 1 milligram of calcium is lost. That means that a 40-gram reduction in animal protein reduces the calcium lost in the urine by 40 milligrams. Assuming about 20 percent of ingested calcium is absorbed, this lowers a person's daily requirement by 200 milligrams. Some experts believe there is no single, universal calcium requirement, but one that is linked to a person's intake of other nutrients, in particular animal proteins and sodium.[22]

Dairy and Bone

For decades, the dairy industry has convincingly marketed milk as the osteoporosis solution. Most baby boomers and their offspring have been indoctrinated into thinking that daily milk is a requirement for the growing body and is the ultimate nutrition. Dairy products are said to provide about 70 percent of the dietary calcium of the United States population.[23]

> *The majority of outcomes showed no significant relationship between consumption of dairy and bone health.*

It can come as a shock to learn that dairy products could actually contribute to bone loss and fracture. Numerous studies published in journals like the American Journal of Public Health suggest that milk is ineffective in preventing osteoporosis. One study compared milk and calcium consumption in 77,000 women over a 12-year period in relation to the incidence of hip and forearm fractures. It found that those with the highest consumption of dairy products *had more fractures* than those who drank less milk. The authors concluded: "These data do not support the hypothesis that higher consumption of milk and other food sources of calcium by adult women protects against hip or forearm fractures."[24] An Australian study examining the dietary history of elderly residents reached the same conclusion, finding that the consumption of milk and cheese in a person at the age of 20 may be linked to an increased rate of hip fracture when that person becomes at risk in old age. [25]

Researchers reviewed 57 studies to determine any correlation between the consumption of dairy foods and bone health. The study found that the majority of outcomes showed no significant relationship between the two. The authors conclude: "The body of scientific evidence appears inadequate to support a recommendation for daily intake of dairy foods to promote bone health in the general U.S. population."[26]

Asia and Osteoporosis

Meanwhile, ignoring conclusive evidence to the contrary, dairy industries in the United States, Europe, Australia, and New Zealand have started promoting dairy consumption to Asian populations. Advertising campaigns assert that dairy consumption will help reverse the pending "epidemic" of osteoporosis in those countries — even though Asian populations boast a much-lower incidence of fragility fracture than Western countries.

Researchers link the rarity of osteoporotic fractures in Asian nations to the Asian diet. The traditional Asian diet is rich in calcium — though not from dairy sources. Most Asian people consume a traditional diet, which includes a diverse range of fresh vegetables, some fruit, soybeans, fresh seafood, and meats. They do not have exposure to refined processed foods, and carbonated drinks, and are not accustomed to eating milk products.

Introducing dairy foods in an attempt to change a diet that has traditionally proven to be beneficial raises many questions, particularly when there is a lack of evidence that it will help to prevent fracture.

Rates of osteoporosis-related fracture are low in Asia, as are rates of breast and prostate cancer. In 1998, the incidence of hip fracture in mainland China was one of the lowest in the world. As Hong Kong has undergone increasing urbanization, hip fractures there have increased to the point of doubling in the last 50 years. The reasons given for this are low calcium, lack of exercise, cigarette smoking, alcoholism, and the increasing use of oral and inhaled steroids.[27] Much of Asian urbanization involves the adoption of Western foods and lifestyle trends. Accordingly, the "Western" diseases of breast and prostate cancer are on the rise in countries like Hong Kong and Singapore. Hong Kong now has three times the rate of breast cancer of mainland China. A study of Japanese women who had immigrated to the United States found that when Western-style diet and lifestyle were adopted, the incidence of estrogen-dependent cancers like breast cancer increased.[28]

A friend of mine, Diane, recently returned from three months of voluntary primary nursing in the villages of southeast Cambodia, near the border with Vietnam. The villagers would queue to see her every day. She reports having seen no evidence of osteoporosis in the elderly population. She also confirms a total lack of dairy product in the diet of these rural people. "Even the buffalo are not milked. The diet is quite simply rice, vegetables and meat. Other than the availability of yogurt in some supermarkets in Phnom Penh, dairy food is not in evidence."

There is Milk, and There is Milk

Milk may not be the healthy food we think it is. A few sobering facts:

- Dairy products, with the exception of skim milk products, are loaded with saturated fat. Fat is directly related to heart disease and cancer.

- Dairy products are also very high in protein, which is linked to calcium loss.

- Insulin-dependent diabetes is linked to dairy products. Studies show a strong correlation between the consumption of dairy products and the incidence of insulin-dependent diabetes.[29]

- Many people are allergic to milk, and others are unable to digest the milk sugar lactose and are lactose intolerant.[30,31]

Because of the artificial, high-pressure environment they are forced to live in, and without their calves, which are slaughtered at birth, milking cows have a high incidence of mastitis and other infections. In her book *Your Life In Your Hands*, Professor Jane Plant points out that "even in the European Union, milk for human consumption can be sold legally even when it contains up to 400,000 somatic pus cells/ml. So one teaspoon of milk can contain 2 million pus cells." [32] For this reason, cows are routinely fed antibiotics. These are then passed directly on to the milk drinkers. A 1990 FDA survey found antibiotics and other drugs in 51 percent of milk samples taken in 14 cities.[33]

For Americans there is an even greater concern. On January 23, 1998, researchers at the Harvard Medical School released a major study providing conclusive evidence that IGF-1 or insulin-like growth factor 1, is a potent risk factor for prostate cancer. The milk of cows injected with synthetic bovine growth hormone (rBGH) to increase milk production has high levels of IGF-1. In his 1996 article in the International Journal of Health Sciences, Dr. Samuel Epstein of the University of Illinois warned of the danger of high levels of IGF-1. He postulated that IGF-1 in rBGH-milk could be a potential risk factor for breast and gastrointestinal cancers as well as prostate cancer.[34] In 1985 the Food and Drug Administration approved the sale of milk from cows treated with rBGH (also known as BST) in large-scale veterinary trials and in 1993 approved commercial sale of milk from rBGH-injected cows. At the same time the FDA prohibited the special labeling of the milk so as to make it impossible for the consumer to distinguish between rBGH and non-rBGH affected milk. Many of the contaminants and risks can be avoided by drinking organic low-fat milk.

Calcium or Not?

Calcium is an essential nutrient. While it is uncertain how much calcium is actually needed, it is certain that diet affects calcium balance. Calcium supplements are not the best way to control osteoporosis for most people. A diet that is modest in protein, high in vegetables, and complemented by exercise is much more effective. Green, leafy vegetables and beans are good sources of calcium that are also moderate in protein and very low in fat. Dark green vegetables, such as broccoli and collard, mustard, and turnip greens are much better sources of calcium than milk. A single cup of broccoli contains almost one-fourth of the U.S. recommended daily amount of calcium. Remember, though, that real requirements may vary depending on the amount of protein and salt that is eaten, and on vitamin D levels. A few minutes of sunlight on the skin every day normally produces all the vitamin D the body needs. People who get little or no sun exposure, or who are older, may need a vitamin D supplement. For more on calcium-rich foods, and food sources of other essential bone nutrients, see Chapter 10.

Calcium is not a stand-alone issue in maintaining bone health. It is not a magic bullet to target and eliminate the disease known as osteoporosis. Bone needs are complex from a nutritional standpoint. Calcium is but one of the needs, and its levels may be very dependent on the rest of the composition of the diet. Focusing just on calcium and assuming that dairy is good for you because it contains calcium is just too simple a solution. It is unfortunately one of the most well-promoted myths in the osteoporosis story.

Section III: Creating Bone Health

✱ 8 ✱

Understanding Health

A holistic approach.

———————

Frail health, more than any other single factor, leads to bone fractures, which is why maintaining good health is fundamental to creating strong bones and preventing fractures later in life. Staying well means more than taking a prescription drug or mineral supplement. The influences on a woman's health are many, and include nutrition and dietary choices, environmental factors, exercise habits, psychological state and genetic makeup. Some influences we have no control over — we each are born with a unique genetic predisposition to certain diseases or health risks. But in the majority of other areas of our lives, we can control our health.

Creating overall health starts from the day we are born, and lasts until the day we die. The air we breath, the water we drink, the food we eat, the amount of exercise we undertake, the amount of sleep we get — all of these things influence our health. When the body is young, it has a tremendous ability to heal and repair; people can get away with ingesting junk food, functioning on little rest, ignoring exercise, drinking too much, and smoking. Such habits don't appear to affect the body too badly. But they do.

> *Every aspect of our health is connected. If one aspect is out of balance, it affects every part of us.*

Once a woman reaches perimenopause, her body quickly lets her know what her limits are, and if she is wise, she will take heed of the signals it gives her. Menopause gives women an opportunity to make significant lifestyle changes in order to stay healthy through the transition and healthy after menopause — mentally, emotionally, and physically. Every aspect of our health is connected, and if one aspect of ourselves is out of balance, then it affects every part of us.

Linda was diagnosed with osteopenia at age 45. She was initially shocked, then worried, especially when her doctor explained that she stood to lose more bone density as she went through menopause. Linda had practiced yoga and meditation all her life, eaten a largely organic, mineral-rich diet, and worked as a physiotherapist, so she was well-informed about the importance of staying flexible and fit. After seeking several opinions and determining that she had no secondary health problems that were contributing to her condition, Linda concluded that she had two choices: Take hormone replacement therapy to further limit bone loss for the duration of the menopause transition, or focus on staying well and fit.

She chose the latter and continued her holistic approach to managing her bone health and her life. She educated herself fully about her options, and what her diagnosis could mean, and understood that there are no predictions, no definitive answers, and no magic-bullet solutions. She decided to take responsibility for her future by doing everything she could to maintain good health. It is now five years since her diagnosis and Linda continues to exercise, eat organic foods, and meditate regularly. She feels very well and has not had a fracture. She no longer feels concerned about her bone density.

The following strategies for a long and healthy life are fundamental to maintaining good bone health and good overall health.

Receiving Adequate Nutrition

Nutrition plays a pivotal role in determining bone health and hip fracture risk. Many elderly people fail to receive adequate intakes of most nutrients, and malnutrition is much worse in those who suffer hip fractures. Several studies have noted that elderly patients, when they are admitted to hospitals with hip fractures, usually have poor nutritional health. A study of 2,500 white women showed that those who had poor nutrition had a significantly higher rate of hip fracture.[1]

Japanese women have the highest life expectancy in the world, as well as a low incidence of breast cancer, heart disease, and hip fractures — a fact many researchers attribute to their low-fat, high-fiber diet rich in minerals, vitamins, anti-oxidants and phytoestrogens (plant substances with estrogen-like effects). Japanese women gain these benefits by consuming an abundance of fresh fruits and vegetables, legumes, whole grains, and seafood.

Maintaining Normal Weight

Some women develop a lifelong tendency to diet, trying to attain a standard of beauty defined by a thin-is-better culture. Many well-controlled studies have shown that when a woman loses weight, regardless of age, she loses bone density.[2] Women who diet and exercise to the point of interrupting their menstrual cycles are also known to lose bone density and even fracture.[3]

Exercise

The importance of exercise cannot be overstated. Weight-bearing exercise increases bone strength and helps the entire body stay fit. A little exercise goes a long way. Walking for 30 minutes three or four times per week can substantially increase bone strength. Exercise will be discussed in greater detail in the following chapter on creating strong bones.

Avoiding Smoking and Alcohol

Smoking damages the bones as well as the heart and lungs. A study of 300 healthy, young women aged 20 to 29 found that smokers had significantly lower spine BMD and a tendency for lower BMD at other sites.[4] According to a 2001 report, postmenopausal women who smoke cigarettes are significantly more likely to sustain a hip fracture than those who don't smoke.[5] Smokers also may absorb less calcium from their diets.[6]

Alcohol has been linked to reduced bone mass because it disrupts the absorption of calcium. The effect is believed to be significant at levels of more than two drinks per day of spirits, beer, or wine. Chronic alcoholism, particularly in men, significantly increases osteoporosis and fractures of the rib, hip, and spine.[7]

However, a French study involving 7,500 women over the age of 75 found that drinking one to three glasses of wine each day may have a positive effect on bone mass. The authors caution that nutritional and physical exercise factors were likely to be involved in the outcome of the study, so it couldn't be entirely attributed to the alcohol.[8]

Job Satisfaction and Personal Happiness

Doing what you love to do in life will bring you happiness, motivation, and probably success. It will also make you energetic and highly resistant to aging and disease. Discovering what you most enjoy, and doing it, is one of the most powerful techniques for a long and healthy life. Medicine acknowledges that our mind and body operate inseparably, and for this reason it makes sense to look for happiness in whatever we pursue.

Happiness has even been shown to cure life-threatening disease. Norman Cousins, a leader in America's intellectual community in 1964, developed the severe condition of ankylosing spondylitis, a painful, progressive, rheumatic disease affecting the spine and other joints, tendons, and ligaments. He had a tremendous will to live and set himself the task of mobilizing all the natural resources of his body and mind to combat the disease. He rejected conventional treatment and instead forged ahead with a self-prescribed regimen built on high doses of both vitamin C and laughter. He enjoyed a steady diet of "Candid Camera" television episodes and Marx Brothers' films. He found that 10 minutes of genuine belly laughter had an anesthetic effect that would give him least two hours of pain-free sleep. Cousins recovered and more than 10 years later wrote about his recovery in a landmark article in The New England Journal of Medicine and a book, *Anatomy of an Illness*.[9] His breakthrough generated an unprecedented interest in mind-body medicine.

Managing Stress

Stress is generated by the tensions and pressures of life. Levels of the stress hormone cortisol produced by the adrenal glands rise when we are under stress, then fall when the stress disappears. But chronic stress, a common phenomenon in Western life, can override our body's natural ability to bounce back. Sustained stress keeps cortisol levels high, which in turn suppresses our immune response.

If we continue to live in stressful circumstances, we are more likely to develop numerous disorders including infections, obesity, poor wound healing, decreased learning and memory skills, hypertension, stroke, heart attacks, and even osteoporosis (low BMD).

High levels of cortisol can result in the extraction of calcium from our bones, and its circulation back into the blood stream. This means that an excess of cortisol will cause bone loss and ultimately could cause fragile bones. Cortisol can directly suppress production of the hormones DHEA and progesterone and can also suppress thyroid activity. These hormones are all involved in regulating bone turnover. Magnesium deficiency could also be a result of stress; magnesium is essential for normal bone metabolism. Adrenaline, which is also released by the adrenal glands when we are stressed, draws magnesium out of the cells and allows it to be flushed out in the urine. [10]

Good health is dependent on managing stress. Research indicates that regular daily exercise, a positive workplace, good friendships, and a spiritual dimension to life are helpful. The practice of meditation is also known to reduce stress levels, improve health and well-being. In a large study published in the Journal of Clinical Psychology in 1989,

Transcendental Meditation was shown to reduce hospital services by 50 percent and reverse biological age by an average of 12 years.

nearly two decades of stress-related research and various meditation and relaxation techniques were compared statistically. Transcendental Meditation (TM) was shown to reduce anxiety twice as much as any other technique.[11] Other studies have revealed that individuals who have been practicing the technique of TM for 20 minutes twice daily for five or more years use hospital services 50 percent less and have an average biological age 12 years younger than their chronological age.[12]

Avoiding Exposure to Chemical Pollution

There is preliminary evidence from two studies — one from Sweden and one from Australia — that exposure to the banned pesticide DDT may affect bone mineral density and possibly increase the risk for fragility fractures. The studies were prompted by research two decades ago that showed DDT affected the fertility of birds and made their eggshells lighter.[13] In the human body, DDT metabolizes into DDE, which is known to affect human hormones. A study of 90 women aged 45 to 65 in northern New South Wales found that those with traces of pesticide in their blood had lower bone density than those with none.[14] A group of 115 men from the general Swedish population, ranging in age from 40 to 75 years old, were similarly tested, and a weak association was found between DDE levels and low bone density.[15]

Because DDT was used widely as a pesticide from the 1950s to the 1970s, these groups of women and men could have been exposed to it at the time when spraying was at its height, and when peak bone mass was being achieved. DDT has a long half-life in the body — about 72 years — so traces are still detectable, even though spraying is no longer permitted in these countries.

The findings of the two initial studies must be confirmed by larger studies. The preliminary research, however, serves as another salutary reminder that hormone-mimicking environmental chemicals (organochlorines) may be harming our health. Organochlorines are also created by motor vehicle emissions, industrial processes and wastes, and pesticides and herbicides. Researchers are finding these chemicals in waterways, soils, and, increasingly, food. Consequently, our bodies are under constant assault from the resulting free radicals (unstable oxygen molecules), which damage cells and are believed to be the root cause of many diseases and chronic illnesses. Since 1980, the incidence of cancer alone has increased by 50 percent in industrialized countries, and from one person in 10 in 1950 to one person in three in 2000. Researchers link the increased incidence of cancer to exposure to carcinogens in the air, water, workplace, or in consumer products.[16]

Some of this damage can be averted through the powerful neutralizing effects of naturally occurring dietary antioxidants or free-radical scavengers in fresh fruits and vegetables, and a supplementation with vitamin C and vitamin E. The consumption of organic foods and avoidance of exposure to chemicals is fundamental to reducing the risk of disease from a toxic environment.

> *Consumption of organic foods and avoidance of exposure to chemicals is fundamental to reducing risk of disease.*

Summary

Creating bone health means creating overall health, not just taking a drug or a nutritional supplement. The following chapters outline what you can do to optimize your health, build strong bones, and avoid fracture. They offer concrete steps you can take if you are concerned about osteoporosis and bone health.

✲ 9 ✲

Positive Reactions

What to do if you have been given a diagnosis of low bone density.

The rush to measure bone density in apparently healthy women has placed many of them in a difficult situation. What do they do when their test results show that they have low bone density? Many physicians accept unquestioningly that a low bone density reading is a precursor to a disabling fracture and reach for their prescription pads, believing this is the best thing they can do for their patients. Chances are, however, that it is not.

For women who have been given a diagnosis of low bone density, the following three steps can help relieve some of the fear and anxiety.

First, find out what the test results mean. What are your actual risks for having a fracture, especially a hip fracture? Perspective helps. Test results are often conveyed in terms of a T-score, a number that rates bone mineral density as compared to a benchmark figure based on healthy, young women in their 20s and 30s — leaving the majority of women with test results that appear abnormal. Instead of looking at your T-score, find out what your Z-score is, a bone mineral density rating based on women your own age. It will give you a more realistic analysis of your bone health. You can also use this information with the questions and tables below to gain an accurate assessment of your risk for hip fracture.

Second, make sure some other medical condition is not causing your low bone density. Some typical tests for this are described below.

Third, take steps to minimize the risk of falling. These steps will do more to prevent hip fractures than any other measure.

Fourth, improve your bone health. You can slow bone loss and increase bone strength without medication, as discussed in Chapter 10.

Whether you are at low risk or high risk, these steps will help your bones and your overall health. Recognize that many well women are diagnosed with osteoporosis or osteopenia based solely on the redefinition of the disease as a measure of low bone density. Bone density, however, is only one aspect of bone strength. Other factors are much more important in determining fracture risk.

Understanding Your Risk of Fracture

Age is an important factor in understanding your risk of fracture. A 50-year-old woman is very unlikely to have a fracture related to osteoporosis, whereas a 90-year-old woman has a 30 percent chance of breaking her hip. Age is an important factor in deciding what your next step will be.

Another important determinant is whether you have had a fracture since your 50th birthday. A personal history of low-trauma fracture is one of the most important risk factors, because it demonstrates that your bones are possibly already fragile, not just that they have the potential to be. "Low trauma" means fracturing a bone with minimal impact. The presence of a spinal fracture is also an important predictor of future fracture.

In assessing risk, family history is a strong determining factor, especially immediate family. If your mother has fractured her hip, that will increase your likelihood of fracture. Other factors also play an important role, such as:

Sedentary Lifestyle — A sedentary lifestyle can cause bone loss. Regular exercise sustains bone remodeling and helps prevent falls in the elderly.

Smoking — Smokers are more at-risk than nonsmokers because of the tendency to have lower bone density, lower body weight, and lower estrogen levels.

Low Body Weight — This is a strong predictor of fracture risk. Research indicates that a weight of 132 pounds or more offers protection. Weight loss is associated with significant BMD loss in postmenopausal women, and many experts advise against constant dieting. Conversely, small bones automatically register lower on bone density tests even if they are not thinner, which can make small bones look more at risk than they are.

Loss of Height — Find out if there has been height loss and how much. Loss of height can be related to compression of discs, but a loss of height of more than 3 centimeters (about 1.2 inches) usually indicates vertebral deformity.

Early or Surgical Menopause — This can cause increased bone loss in some women.

Cessation of Periods — If your period has stopped for 12 months or more (other than because of pregnancy), you may be at greater risk. Eating disorders, overexercising, and emotional trauma may interfere with normal menstruation. This can influence bone remodeling and cause reduced bone density

Prescription Medications — Certain drugs like corticosteroids are associated with bone loss and increased rate of fracture. (See full list of drugs at the end of Chapter 4.)

Certain diseases that cause frequent diarrhea are associated with osteoporosis, such as celiac disease or Crohn's disease.

Understanding the factors that can increase your risk of fracture will help you to put your test results in perspective. Another way of doing this is to try to quantify your risk, as the next section explains.

Assessing Your Risk of Hip Fracture

Hip fractures are the most debilitating fractures — and should therefore be the target of preventative strategies. Assessing your actual risk of hip fracture can determine whether you need to be concerned and consider aggressive treatment, or whether your risks are minimal and you can rest at ease.

A 1995 study published in the New England Journal of Medicine followed more than 9,000 women to determine which risk factors are significant in determining a risk for hip fracture.[1] The results showed that bone density was only one of several factors that have to be taken into account, and that low bone density only became a cause for concern in the presence of a least five other risk factors. The factors that significantly contributed to hip fracture risk are outlined below. To approximate your actual risk of hip fracture, put a check by the risk factors you have and total the number of checks.

1. Age greater than 80.	☐
2. History of hip fracture in your mother.	☐
3. Any fracture (except hip fracture) since age 50.	☐
4. Fair, poor, or very poor health (as opposed to good or excellent health).	☐
5. Previous history of hyperthyroidism.	☐
6. Taking seizure medication.	☐
7. Taking long-acting tranquilizers (benzodiazepenes).	☐
8. Current weight less than it was at age 25.	☐
9. Height at age 25 greater than 5 feet 6 inches tall.	☐
10. Caffeine intake more than the equivalent of two cups of coffee per day.	☐
11. On feet 4 hours a day or less.	☐
12. Do not walk for exercise.	☐
13. Cannot rise from a chair without using your arms.	☐
14. Poor depth perception – the ability to see objects in perspective.	☐
15. Difficulty seeing contrasts.	☐
16. Resting pulse rate is greater than 80 beats per minute.	☐
TOTAL _____	

After you have determined your number of risk factors, use this information together with your bone density testing results (your Z-scores, if you have them) to get an approximation of your risk. If you are not sure where your testing results fall, ask your health-care provider whether your results fall in the lowest, middle, or upper third *for women your age.* The chart below determines the percent of women like you who will have a hip fracture within the next 10 years, when they become 72.*

Estimated percent of women who will have a hip fracture within the next 10 years, starting at age 72*.

HIGHEST THIRD BONE DENSITY (Z-score >= 0.43)
If your bone density is in the highest third for women your age, and your number of risk factors is:

0 - 2:	Your risk is 1.1 percent
3 - 4:	Your risk is 1.9 percent
5 or greater:	Your risk is 9.4 percent

MIDDLE THIRD (AVERAGE) BONE DENSITY (Z-score -0.42 to +0.42)
If your bone density is in the middle third for women your age, and your number of risk factors is:

0 - 2:	Your risk is 1.1 percent
3 - 4:	Your risk is 5.6 percent
5 or greater:	Your risk is 14.7 percent

LOWEST THIRD BONE DENSITY (Z-score <= - 0.43)
If your bone density is in the lowest third for women your age, and your number of risk factors is:

0 - 2:	Your risk is 2.6 percent
3 - 4:	Your risk is 4.0 percent
5 or greater:	Your risk is 27.3 percent

---

*The study participants had an average age of 72. The following chart can be used as an approximation only, because the study group may have different characteristics from you. In addition, the original data was reported as annual risk per 1,000 women-years, and has been transformed to percent risk per 10 years to make the approximation of risk more easily understood.

Suppose you have a Z-score of -0.2 (middle third) and you have two risk factors — your height is greater than 5 feet 6 inches and your resting pulse rate is 82 beats per minute. From the chart, you can see that your risk of fracture is 1.1 percent. If you were to take drugs to increase your bone density to the highest third, your risk for fracture would not change. To greatly reduce the risk of fracture, people need to reduce the number of risk factors. People who have five or more risk factors need to consider making lifestyle changes to improve their health. Many of the risk factors, such as "not walking for exercise," can be changed without medications. Note also that bone density doesn't play a major role until a person has *five or more* risk factors.

In assessing your osteoporosis risk, other factors may also need to be taken into account. For example, if you smoke or take medications like corticosteroids, your risk is increased. If you have had an early menopause or surgical menopause, your risk may also be increased.

Checking for Other Causes

If your bone density is very low (or even if your bone density is normal), and you want to eliminate other risk factors, then ask your doctor for the following tests:

- If you have lost height and if your DXA scan shows low BMD in the spine, then a lateral spine X-ray will determine whether there has been any compression fracturing.

- Blood (serum) vitamin D and calcium levels.

- A thyroid test — especially if there is a family history of hypothyroidism or hyperthyroidism.

- A 24-hour calcium/urine test will measure how much calcium is being lost in the urine. If there are high levels of calcium in the urine, then you need to see a specialist.

- DXA scan in more than one bone site. It is possible that there can be some inaccuracies with DXA scanning, particularly if you have already had a spinal fracture that has caused some compression in your vertebrae. This can make your bones seem denser than they are. Sometimes, fractures of the vertebrae go unnoticed, as they can be painless. Measuring the hip as well can give a more accurate reading.

- A bone marker urine test can gauge the approximate rate of bone breakdown or bone resorption by measuring the breakdown products of collagen. It is normally quite high postmenopause, but repeat testing every three to six months will indicate whether bone loss is occurring. The tests to request are Dpd, or deoxypyridinoline, and NTx, or N-telopeptide, which measure bone breakdown or resorption, and bone alkaline phosphatase (ALP), which measures bone formation.

- Celiac disease. There are three antibody blood tests which, if all are positive, indicate a high probability of celiac disease. The tests are: endomysial, reticulin (IgA), and gliadin (IgG and IgA) antibodies.

- For men, serum testosterone levels could also be measured.

- Have blood levels of magnesium, zinc, manganese, boron, and other trace minerals tested.

Preventing Falls

As we age, muscle mass naturally decreases, skin becomes thinner, and fat shifts to the center of the body — physical changes that decrease the body's ability to pad itself in the event of a fall and prevent fractures. Therefore, regardless of bone density, people must take extra care to avoid falls as they age. Studies show that fall-prevention strategies significantly reduce the incidence of hip fractures. The following steps can help reduce the risk of falling:

1. Maintain a Safe Home
The home can be a hazardous place. Many falls occur as a result of obstacles such as loose floor rugs and mats, electrical cords, and poorly placed furniture.

Suggestions:

- Have your home assessed for risk by an occupational therapist.
- Install handrails around steps and stairs, in the bathroom by the shower and toilet, and outside at any entrance to your house.
- Cover steps and stairs with nonslip material.
- Remove all loose rugs, and secure carpets with nonskid tape.
- Do not polish or wax floors.
- Remove extension cords.
- Clear clutter so that you can move easily from room to room.
- Arrange furniture such as coffee tables so you can move around easily.
- Check that lighting is adequate and effective.
- Install an emergency response system.
- Have telephone extensions in each main area.
- Use a cordless telephone where possible.

The bathroom is the most dangerous room in the house. Suggestions:

- Remove loose bathmats.
- Use nonskid mats, abrasive strips, and grab bars in showers and tubs.
- Ensure lighting is adequate.
- Make sure toilet seats are not wobbly and are high enough.

The kitchen is the second-most dangerous room. Suggestions:

- Ensure lighting is more than adequate.
- Rearrange cupboards so that you don't have to reach or bend far for commonly used items.
- Put appliance cords well out of the way.
- Use a sturdy step stool with handrails.
- Clean up spills from floors immediately.

Bedroom, living room, and hallway floors are dangerous areas with many minor dangers that can become major hazards. Suggestions:

- Remove clutter.
- Remove loose mats and rugs.
- Have bright lights in stairways and hallways.
- Install strong handrails running the length of halls and stairs.
- Raise beds and chairs to a height that is easy to get into and out of.
- Remove caster wheels from furniture.
- Have a bedside lamp that is easy to reach and turn on.
- Install a night light.
- Have telephone within easy reach of bed.
- Watch out for pets — they can get underfoot and cause a fall.

2. Understand the Side Effects of Any Medication You Take

Certain medications such as sedatives, antidepressants, and antipsychotic drugs can cause dizziness, drowsiness, and blurred vision, which can lead to falling. Medications can also reduce alertness, affect balance and gait, and cause a sudden drop in blood pressure when standing or rising from a chair. People taking multiple medications are at greater risk of falling. Suggestions:

- Discuss the side effects and interactions of your medications with your physician or pharmacist.
- Request the lowest effective dose.
- If you see more than one physician, make sure that each one knows all the medication you are taking.
- Take all your medications with you when you visit the doctor.
- Get rid of all out-of-date medications.
- Make sure all medications are clearly labeled and stored in a well-lit area.
- Use walking aids, if using medications that affect balance.

- Get up slowly when lying down or sitting up if you have heart problems or high blood pressure.

- Talk to your doctor about managing poor bladder control to avoid rushing to the restroom.

- Limit alcohol intake. Drinking can make you unsteady and it can interact with medications.

3. Maintain Your Eyesight

Poor vision is associated with an increased risk for falling. Suggestions:

- Have annual checkups with your eye doctor to monitor for conditions such as glaucoma and cataracts.

- Keep eyeglasses clean.

- Add contrasting color strips to handrails and steps in the home.

4. Wear Sturdy Footwear and Reduce Environmental Hazards

- Wear low-heeled, supportive shoes with rubber soles.

- Avoid loose slippers, shoes with leather soles, or high heels.

- Never walk in your stocking feet.

- Avoid uneven walking surfaces, broken or cracked sidewalks, and construction areas.

- Park your car where it is clear of snow and ice.

- Avoid wet surfaces.

- Install sensor lights outdoors that will turn on whenever there is motion.

5. Wear Hip Protectors

Thinner and frail women have less fat and soft tissue to protect them when they fall. Elderly people who are at high risk for fracture can wear a padded undergarment to absorb the energy of a high-impact fall and reduce the risk of hip fracture. There is evidence that the pads can reduce hip fracture rates by half.

Check out the following resources, if you are interested in further reading:

Tremblay, K.R. Jr., Barber, C.E. "Preventing Falls in the Elderly." Colorado State University Cooperative Extension. http://www.ext.colostate.edu/pubs/consumer/10242.html

American Academy of Orthopaedic Surgeons. For a free brochure on fall prevention, call 1-800-824-BONES (2663). http://orthoinfo.aaos.org/

Taking Positive Action to Create Bone Health

Many of the risk factors for fractures involve lifestyle choices that you can control and modify. The next chapter explains how to decrease your risks, and take positive action to increase bone density and create better health.

❋ 10 ❋

Creating Strong Bones

What every woman should know.

My parents lead very active lives and keep excellent health. They are both in their 80s and are inspiring examples of how meaningless a diagnosis of osteoporosis can be. They maintain a large property, grow their own vegetables, and my mother has a beautiful flower garden. They walk daily for exercise, and are actively involved in various community projects. They take great interest in each member of our large, extended family, and are very supportive of us all. My mother broke her wrist in her 60s, but apart from that has never fractured. She is organized, has good physical stamina, and keeps her days full; sometimes I think she has more energy than I do. She also has been the "eyes" for two people since my father lost his sight 15 years ago as the result of a blood clot.

My father served in the New Zealand army medical corps in Italy and Egypt during World War II and has been physically fit all his life. He has never fractured. He is a strong swimmer and was president of the town swimming club for many years. For 65 years, he has been closely associated with a large rural camp facility, built originally for the local church youth, and now used mostly for outdoor education of the region's school children. Although he is soon to retire after 50 years as chairman of the camp trust, my father volunteers many days there working on, maintaining, and upgrading the property.

Obviously, his bones can withstand the constant demands he makes of them. He lifts wheelbarrows of concrete, digs ditches, climbs ladders, plants trees, and finds no task too daunting, despite his blindness. Recently he helped design an obstacle course involving challenging physical activities, such as rope ladders and a rope bridge. The latest addition is a steep, 20-meter slide that is not for the fainthearted. On a recent visit, my father demonstrated how quickly an 86- year-old could travel on highly polished stainless steel. I watched, heart in mouth, as he hurtled the length of the slide, somersaulted off the end, and lay laughing in a heap, quipping that the advantage of being blind is that you can't see the end coming.

When I look at my parents and the active lives that they lead, I see them exemplifying the way in which simple lifestyle choices can help people live longer, healthier, and happier lives. Exercising on a regular basis and eating healthy foods are two of the best ways to maintain good health and create excellent bone health.

Exercise

Study after study shows that moderate exercise helps to prevent a host of chronic illnesses, from diabetes to heart disease — even, in many cases, osteoporosis. Exercise benefits the skeleton, and is the single most effective strategy to prevent fragility fracture. No other agent, hormonal or mineral, can actually cause the skeleton to become heavier or sturdier in response to the demands made of it. Bone formation is stimulated by the mechanical forces that exercise generates, particularly higher-impact activities like jogging, running, and jumping that generate more effect on bones than lower-impact exercise like swimming or walking.

The force of muscles pulling against bones promotes new bone growth, and the more you use your muscles, the more this stimulates bone remodeling and bone formation. This effect has been repeatedly observed in athletes. A recent study of volleyball players demonstrated that top male volleyball players show remarkably high bone density in the hip and spine regions, and high bone density in their arms and legs. Interestingly, the arm used to spike the volleyball was up to 9 percent more dense than the less-involved arm, believed to be a result of the body's adaptation to the greater demands made on that arm.[1]

> *Exercise prevented or reversed about 1 percent of bone loss per year at the spine and the hip.*

A review of all the randomized controlled studies done on exercise and bone mass in pre- and postmenopausal women concluded that exercise prevented or reversed about 1 percent of bone loss per year at the spine and the hip.[2] There is also evidence that women with the lowest BMD tend to show the greatest response to exercise — a great incentive for anyone with a BMD diagnosis of osteoporosis.[3]

When it comes to exercise, age is no barrier. People more than 80 years old can reduce their risk of osteoporosis while also improving muscle tone and balance.[4] Exercise programs offered by trained health professionals that target strength and balance, or strength and endurance, have been found to reduce the frequency of falls in high-risk, older people. These specific exercise programs incorporate walking, the gentle and gradual use of weights, and exercises to increase balance. A New Zealand home exercise program delivered by trained nurses to 450 women and men aged 79 to 94 resulted in a 30 percent reduction in the incidence of falls.[5] Interestingly, the study found no decrease in the incidence of fracture.

Coincidentally, my father participated in this program. He followed the exercise routines daily for several months and significantly increased the amount of weight he could lift and the duration of use. Soon after the program ended, he underwent a major surgical procedure. His excellent recovery could in part be attributed to the level of strength and fitness achieved at the time.

Physical activity is one of the most important factors in acquiring peak bone mass during youth. Many researchers believe that as children and young adults log increasing numbers of hours watching television and sitting in front of computers, their bone mass may be suffering for it. High impact exercise has been found to have the most beneficial effect on bone mass in girls before puberty, rather than after.[6]

Regular exercise has numerous other benefits. It increases well-being and fitness. It also helps protect against conditions like heart disease, cancer, depression, and Alzheimer's disease.[7] In addition, weight training can give a sense of competency when daily tasks such as lifting, carrying groceries, or pushing the lawn mower become much easier. Although weight training is not aerobic, it helps increase metabolism, which can help shed excess weight.

Sedentary Lives

Lack of exercise and immobility will reduce bone density, general strength, and fitness. Bedridden patients lose muscle and bone, and have increased levels of urinary calcium, indicating that calcium is being lost from the bone.

A recent survey of adult New Zealanders revealed that they spend an average of 40 minutes a day on grooming, an hour and a half socializing, an hour and a half eating, two hours watching TV and eight minutes exercising.[8] Most likely this is similar throughout the developed nations. Life in the 21st century works against us being physically active. In fact, it continues to get easier to avoid exercising. Daily activity is geared toward working our bodies less and less, as technology replaces physical effort. Many of us sit for hours in front of computer terminals and now send much of our mail electronically — threatening to deny us even the walk to the mailbox. We drive from destination to destination — no matter how short the drive; and when we arrive there, escalators and elevators lift us from floor to floor.

The National Aeronautics and Space Administration physicians discovered astronauts lost bone in space at the dizzying rate of 1.5 percent per month. Dr. Norman Thagard spent 115 days in space on the Russian space station Mir. He lost 11.7 percent of his bone density and 17.5 pounds of overall muscle and weight during his sojourn. Most of this loss came from the hip and lower spine. Dr. Frank M. Sulzman, director of life science research at NASA, says a trip to Mars, which is estimated to take between one and two years each way, may leave an astronaut permanently crippled upon return to Earth.[9]

No group is at higher risk for depression, disease, and early death than people who are completely sedentary. Studies from the Russian space program also showed that young cosmonauts subjected to the forced inactivity of space flight fell prey to depression. When they were put on a schedule of regular exercise, the depression was avoided.[10]

Exercise and the Older Person

Physiologists used to believe that exercise primarily benefited us at young ages when muscles are in their prime developmental stage. However, research with the elderly has conclusively demonstrated that a person can take up exercise at any age — even centenarians will receive the same increase in strength, stamina, and muscle mass. Weight training, in particular, has special benefits for the frail elderly. In a 1992 study of frail, very old volunteers who were prone to falling easily, Maria Fiatarone and colleagues at the Hebrew Rehabilitation Center for Aged observed that, after adopting a regular resistance training program, men and women tripled their thigh muscle mass and dramatically lowered their risk of falls.[11]

In 1990, researchers from Tufts University showed that elderly nursing home residents, ranging in age from 86 to 96, dramatically increased their strength and improved their balance after just eight weeks of supervised weight training. Now studies have proved that working out with free weights or machines can help restore lost bone density, as well as reduce knee pain from arthritis and keep the body sensitive to the insulin it produces to keep sugar levels in balance.[12]

A recent study indicates that regular exercise may also reduce the risk of developing Alzheimer's disease. The study examined the long-term health habits of 373 people — 126 of them with Alzheimer's disease and 247 of them without. The patients with Alzheimer's disease had had lower levels of physical activity earlier in life.[13]

Exercise also reduces the need for medications such as antihypertensives, antidepressants, and hypnotics that can alter balance and coordination and result in a fall.[14] There are four main types of exercise outlined below.

1. Aerobic

Aerobic exercise increases cardiovascular function and strength. Walking is great aerobic exercise that stimulates the leg and hip bones by the impact of your feet hitting the ground. There is, however, little or no evidence that aerobic exercise alone will increase bone density.

2. Flexibility

Stretching exercises promote flexibility, which helps to prevent falls. Having strong and flexible joints also means that you are less likely to suffer joint injuries. Yoga is excellent in this regard. It is weight-bearing exercise, and in the various yoga postures, the muscles pull on the bone stimulating further remodeling.

3. Balance Training

As we age our sense of balance becomes less, and as a consequence, we are more at risk of falling. Balance training occurs in Tai Chi or other programs specially designed to improve balance.

Visit a local park in the early morning in China and you will see older men and women practicing Tai Chi, a series of postures and exercises characterized by slow, relaxing, and graceful movements. Tai Chi enhances balance and body awareness. Legend has it that in the 12th century, a group of Chinese monks decided to try a new form of meditation — one that would imitate the rhythms of the world and the life all around them. Tai Chi was the result.

> *The most notable outcome of a study of Tai Chi was a 47.5 percent reduction in the rate of multiple falls. Fear of falling was also reduced.*

The main principle of Tai Chi is that it uses subtle movements that cause energy to flow in the body. Tai Chi, according to traditional Chinese medicine, is an excellent way of accumulating energy (chi), storing it, and then circulating it through the body. This balances the body and prevents and heals disease. Studies show that Tai Chi can improve strength, flexibility, and endurance in patients suffering from osteoarthritis. It is an excellent weight-bearing exercise, which can decrease joint swelling and tenderness, improve balance, and reduce the incidence of falls in men and women over 70 years old.[15]

It is one of the only exercises that teaches how to bear all the body weight on one leg at a time. This promotes increased bone formation in the weight-bearing pelvic bones and femur. A U.S. study of the effect of regular Tai Chi exercises over a 15-week period included

200 participants age 70 and older. The participants were divided into groups for Tai Chi, balance training, and education. The most notable outcome was a 47.5 percent reduction in the rate of multiple falls for the Tai Chi group. Fear of falling was also reduced. The groups receiving balance training and education did not have significantly lower rates of falling.[16]

Commentators at the time noted that the success of Tai Chi is a reminder that relatively "low tech" approaches should not be overlooked in the search for ways to prevent disability and maintain physical performance in late life. And it needn't take a lot of time — a mere 10 minutes of Tai Chi practice a day is reported to be beneficial for most people who choose this exercise as a part of their health regimen. Once you have received qualified instruction, you can practice it successfully at home, or in your local park!

4. Resistance or Strength Training

Many studies confirm that strength training by using weights and high-impact exercises can build bone. As muscles contract when we lift weights, they pull on the bone to which they are attached, which then stimulates the bone to build in that area. For this reason is it important to practice a range of exercises that will stimulate the whole skeleton, particularly those areas at higher risk for fracture.

All four types of exercise are important in maintaining fitness, good health, and preventing osteoporosis. But for exercise to be most effective in preventing or slowing bone loss, it must stress the skeleton. As long as exercise does not involve any sudden or excessive strain on the bones and is compatible with a person's general health, then the more exercise the better, from a skeletal point of view. Many experts recommend that people alternate their exercise routine so that the muscles (and bone) receive a varied workout. The idea is that if you can surprise the bone in the way you load it, you may continue to stimulate more bone mineralization and bone strengthening.

A heavier weight lifted fewer times is better than a lighter load lifted more often. A 1996 exercise study compared two types of strength training regimens, which differed in the number of repetitions and the weights lifted. The strength program that involved heavy amounts of weight with low repetitions significantly increased bone density at the hip and forearm sites, whereas the endurance program that featured lighter amounts of weight and high numbers of repetitions had no effect.[17] Strength training is also important for maintaining muscle strength with aging.

Weight training isolates specific muscle groups in various parts of your body — shoulders, chest, arms, back, legs, and stomach — and works them one at a time. A variety of exercises are available for each muscle group. Most experts recommend that you establish a routine that works all of the different muscle groups at least once during the course of a week. It is also advisable to change your weight-training routine periodically by trying new exercises that will work the muscles in a slightly different way. The following weight-training exercises that cover all the muscle groups are suggested for healthy adults.[18] It is important always to learn safe lifting techniques. Ask an expert to teach you how to do them.

• Biceps curl	• Bench press
• Overhead press	• Leg press
• Wrist curl	• Half squats
• Reverse wrist curl	• Hip abduction/adduction
• Triceps extension	• Hamstring curl
• Forearm pronation/supination	• Hip flexion
	• Hip extension

It is important to understand that a woman's body will respond differently to weight training than a man's because of hormonal differences. The hormone testosterone plays a major role in muscular development. Because women have less of this hormone, they tend not to "bulk-up" with weight training.

How To Get Started

The first word of advice on lifting weights is: "Proceed with caution." It's essential to begin with very light weights — weights that are so easy to lift they seem to be flying through the air. Don't try to prove yourself. Strength comes with time and practice; lifting heavy amounts of weight too early in your regimen can lead to injuries that prevent you from exercising at all.

It's best to follow a routine developed by a qualified training expert who can also demonstrate technique and form. Gyms and health clubs usually have on-site trainers. Many fitness consultants can be hired privately. For the budget-conscious, a trip to the library can be helpful; there is no shortage of fitness books that feature explanations and photos of many exercises. Web sites can also help you get started with your weight-training program.

Miriam Nelson's book *Strong Women Strong Bones* (Lothian Books 2000) has an excellent exercise program that you can do at home — whether you are just starting to exercise, or are a pro. Her book subscribes to many of the osteoporosis myths, and should therefore be read selectively. But it contains good nutritional advice, and is an excellent source for anyone who wants to do weight training at home.

She also has a Web site *www.strongwomen.com* and for a fee will provide you with a personalized exercise program.

General Rules for Resistance Training

- Consult your health-care provider before beginning any new exercise program.
- A warm-up is essential and will help prevent injury. Walking in place, stepping, or jumping rope for a few minutes will help get your muscles geared up for action.
- Go slowly. Start with light weights and lift them slowly, in a controlled manner. Do not strain.
- Most experts recommend that you exercise larger muscles groups before smaller ones to achieve maximum benefits. To strengthen the legs, for example, work the quadriceps muscles before the calf muscles.
- Use the same amount of weight in your left and right hands. Even if one side of your body seems to be stronger, be consistent in the amount of weights you use.
- Don't overtrain. Rest one or two days before exercising the same muscle group a second time.
- Follow the workout instructions and guidelines about the number of times to lift each weight (repetitions), and how many sets of each exercise to do.
- Don't forget to breathe! Keep your muscles oxidized.
- Stretch at the completion of your workout to help avoid stiffness and injury.

Precautions

It is extremely important that anyone who undertakes strength training is properly supervised to ensure good technique, especially if they have low bone mass. Weight training may be dangerous if performed improperly or without supervision. If you already have osteoporosis, or have had a fragility fracture, it is very important that you avoid high-impact weight lifting, jumping, abrupt or explosive movements, twisting movements, and intense abdominal exercises. Individuals with high blood pressure, back problems, or hernias should consult a physician prior to engaging in a weight-training program.

How Often Should You Exercise?

Most studies show that people who exercise for one hour, two to three times a week, can significantly slow or prevent bone loss — a benefit equivalent to that achieved by people who exercise every day.[19] Experts recommend easing yourself into an exercise program and gradually increasing your routine over time. For elderly or sedentary people, exercise should be gradually introduced to minimize fatigue and sore muscles. It is also important to have variety in the program and make sure that all muscle groups are being exercised. A carefully supervised strength-training program can do that.

Adding weights to the body during aerobic exercise is an excellent way to do at least two forms of exercise simultaneously. Ankle and arm weights that can be purchased for little investment can be worn for short periods during light exercise.

Exercise Summarized

> *Exercise is the single most important strategy to maintain healthy bones.*

Exercise is the single most important strategy to maintain healthy bones. For exercise to be effective, it must be continued throughout life. If we are immobile or inactive, it will lead to bone loss. Sustained weight-bearing exercise will maintain bone formation and help prevent fracture. Older people who walk and exercise regularly have better coordination, muscle strength, and flexibility — important factors in preventing falls. While exercise is the most important strategy for maintaining healthy bone, dietary and nutritional factors also play a significant role.

Dietary and Nutritional Factors

Diet has a significant effect on bone health, which makes sense, considering the process by which bone is constantly being dissolved and rebuilt involves various nutrients and minerals extracted from the blood supply. Yet, achieving the optimum dietary intake of essential nutrients may not be as easy as eating an apparent "balanced diet."

Many high-protein foods — including meat, eggs, and dairy products — contain rich sources of phosphoric and sulfuric acid. The consumption of such foods, known as "acid ash" foods, will cause acid to form in the body and over time will alter the body's pH balance — which measures the degree of acidity or alkalinity in the blood. As the pH level becomes acidic, the body buffers this by leaching calcium from the bone. Even a small drop in the body's pH can cause a dramatic increase in bone loss.[20]

Because of this, it is important to eat foods that are alkaline. Increasing your intake of alkaline-producing foods — leafy greens, sea vegetables, nonstarchy vegetables, nuts and seeds — will create a bone-nutrient rich, pH balancing diet that reduces cal-

> *Even a small drop in the body's pH can cause a dramatic increase in bone loss.*

cium excretion and bone loss. It can also limit the need for supplements, as these foods are a rich source of vitamins, minerals, and protein. Sea vegetables (seaweeds), for example, contain high amounts of calcium, phosphorus, magnesium, boron, iron, iodine, and sodium.

An investigation of the diets of elderly men and women in Framingham, Massachusetts, found that people who ate more fruits and vegetables rich in potassium and magnesium had less bone mass loss in the hip and forearm than those elderly people who ate less of these foods.[21] A follow-up study also found that high fruit and vegetable intake appears to be protective in men, and a high candy consumption is associated with low bone mass in both men and women.[22]

Protein is also important for bone health, and too little can have an adverse effect on bone. People's protein needs vary, depending on body mass and activity level. Adults are recommended to have approximately 40 to 60 grams of protein daily. Meat, fish, eggs, and milk have large quantities of protein. Vegetable protein is found in grains such as rice and wheat, beans, lentils, nuts and seeds. Pumpkin, squash, and sunflower seeds contain high amounts of protein. They are also most nutritious eaten raw. Flaxseeds and sesame seeds are high in protein and also a good source of calcium. Walnuts, almonds and cashews are the highest in protein of the commonly eaten nuts. Lentils have a lot of protein, while soybeans contain more than twice as much protein as other beans. Other high-protein legumes include garbanzos and black beans.

> *Many experts recommend reducing meat and dairy intake, and increasing vegetable protein consumption.*

Interestingly, the source of protein can affect bone strength. The Study of Osteoporotic Fracture (SOF) trial showed that women who consumed more animal protein than vegetable protein had a higher rate of bone loss at the hip. It also showed a greater risk of hip fracture in women who consumed more animal protein than women who ate vegetable protein.[23]

Many experts therefore recommend reducing meat and dairy intake, and increasing vegetable protein consumption.

> *When animal proteins were eliminated from the diet, calcium losses were cut in half.*

When meat protein consumption is high, then more calcium is required as well. A 1994 report in the American Journal of Clinical Nutrition showed that when animal proteins were eliminated from the diet, calcium losses were cut in half.[24] Another study followed more than 85,000 American women for 12 years. Those who ate the most animal protein (meat, poultry and dairy) had a significantly higher risk of osteoporotic fractures.[25]

Phytoestrogens

Phytoestrogens are plant compounds that have a multitude of hor-mone-like properties that may be beneficial to women. There is growing evidence that regular consumption of fruits, vegetables, grains, and legumes rich in these plant hormones can positively influ-ence a woman's health and hormone balance. Phytoestrogen-rich foods may decrease menopause symptoms including hot flashes, help prevent osteoporosis, and reduce the incidence of heart dis-ease.[26,27,28] The relationship, if any, between phytoestrogens and estrogen-sensitive cancers like breast and prostate has yet to be researched definitively. The incidence of such cancers is low in Asian communities with a soy-based diet.[29,30] Soy is a concentrated source of phytoestrogens.

The traditional diets of approximately half the world's population contain moderate to high levels of phytoestrogens. In Asian cultures, women traditionally have a diet that is low fat, high fiber, and rich in a wide variety of fresh fruit and vegetables (phytoestrogens). This stands in contrast to the high-protein, carbohydrate-rich, fat-based diet more typically found in Western countries. A study of Japanese women who had immigrated to the United States found that when Western-style diet and lifestyle was adopted, the incidence of estro-gen-dependent cancers, like breast cancer, increased.[31]

There is increasing evidence that soy, in particular, has an effect on bone density, but there is no evidence for fracture prevention. A Hong Kong study of 130 women, aged 30 to 40, indicated that a high soy intake appears to reduce the rate of bone mineral density decline in premenopausal Chinese women. Women consuming the highest amount of soy had the lowest rate of bone loss.[32] A similar study of 85 Japanese women also indicated that high soy protein intake is associated with a higher bone mineral density, and a lower level of bone resorption. The authors noted that further studies are needed to confirm just how soy has this effect.[33]

Bacteria in the intestine transform phytoestrogens into active compounds in the bloodstream that are similar to a weak type of estrogen. Some individuals may lack the necessary bacteria to make this conversion. Antibiotics can also reduce the effect.

Phytoestrogens are found in:

Soy — tofu, tempeh, miso, soy milk, soy flour and roasted soybeans, and soy extract powders
Legumes — chickpeas, lentils, and many beans including mung, haricot, broad, kidney, and lima
Wholegrain Cereals — wheat, wheat germ, barley, rye, rice, bran, oats
Fruit — cherries, apples, pears, peaches, apricots, plums and other stone fruit, and rhubarb
Seeds — linseed or flaxseed, sunflower, anise, sesame
Vegetables — green and yellow vegetables, carrots, fennel, onion, garlic
Vegetable Oils — olive oil
Herbs and Roots — ginseng, licorice, hops

Soy is Controversial

These days, traditional methods of soy preparation involving a long process of fermentation have been abandoned in favor of a quicker form of processing. Soy milk, for example, is produced by soaking the beans in an alkaline solution, then heating them to about 115 degrees Celsius. This produces difficult-to-digest proteins and phytates that can block the essential uptake of minerals. It appears that the traditional methods of preparation reduced soy's mineral-robbing "anti-nutrients," and improved its digestibility. The only modern, commercial soy foods that undergo this fermentation are tempeh (not tofu) and miso (not soy sauce). While traditionally prepared tofu may be on the market, as of yet, there is no distinct labeling to mark it as such.

Soy is also being genetically engineered to be resistant to herbicides, and now floods the global market in its altered form. Genetically engineered foods have been controversial because the effect of this altered genetic material on humans is unknown and untested. To avoid consuming genetically engineered soy, it is necessary to eat products labeled "organic," "GE free," or "No GMOs."

Some experts warn against feeding soy milk to infants, as large quantities of even weak plant hormone may be inappropriate for children. The effect of adding large quantities of soy (particularly soy milk) to the adult diet is also unknown. Some people speculate that because soy foods are relatively new to Western men and women, their digestive systems may not have evolved to cope with them.

Other Dietary Considerations

Sodium (salt)

A definite link between salt intake and fracture risk has not yet been established, though increases in dietary salt have led to an increase in the loss of calcium in the urine. People who reduce their sodium intake to 1 to 2 grams per day cut their calcium requirement by an average of 60 milligrams per day.[34] Most nutrition experts therefore recommend less salt and less highly salted foods.

Caffeine

Most nutritional experts recommend avoiding coffee or restricting consumption to one cup a day. Coffee is acidic and is therefore linked to increased bone loss, but there is no evidence that it is linked to fragility fractures. In one trial, caffeine was linked with lower bone mass, but only in women who consumed relatively little calcium.[35] The authors of this report conclude that two to three cups of coffee per day might speed bone loss in women with calcium intakes of less than 800 milligrams per day.

Vitamin D

Sometimes called a hormone and sometimes a nutrient, vitamin D helps to control the formation of bone tissue. It increases the amount of calcium and phosphorus the body absorbs from the small intestine, and thus helps regulate the growth, hardening, and repair of the bones. Vitamin D is essential for the normal growth and development of the teeth, bones, and cartilage in children. It's also needed to keep adult teeth in good repair. Vitamin D also prevents osteomalacia, or rickets, a deficiency disease characterized by malformations of bones and teeth in children, and by brittle, easily broken bones in adults. Age-related vitamin D deficiency leads to malabsorption of calcium, accelerated bone loss, and increased risk for hip fracture. Vitamin D supplementation with calcium has been found to retard bone loss and reduce hip fracture.[36]A recent analysis demonstrated that calcium and vitamin D supplementation is a cost-effective strategy to decrease vertebral fracture risk in women with corticosteroid-induced osteopenia.[37]

A randomized controlled United Kingdom trial of 2,686 men and women 65 to 85 years old found that supplementing with oral vitamin D every four months over the course of five years reduced the rate of fracture. The authors conclude that supplementation every four months with 100,000 IU oral vitamin D may prevent fractures without adverse effects — for as little as $2 annually.[38]

There are two forms of vitamin D: ergocalciferol, which is found in a relatively small selection of foods such as herring, mackerel, salmon, and halibut; and cholecalciferol, which the body manufactures when exposed to the sun. Vitamin D is fat-soluble, can build up in the body, and therefore is highly toxic when taken in large doses for a long time. Low vitamin D levels can be determined from a blood test.

The most important source of vitamin D is sunlight exposure of the skin. Severe vitamin D deficiency is therefore prevalent among people who have insufficient exposure to the sun, including many elderly people who may be institutionalized or confined indoors. A study of veiled Muslim women living in Denmark found that the women needed to supplement with at least three times the recommended daily amount of the vitamin to secure a normal level of 25-hydroxy-vitamin D, the metabolite of vitamin D that circulates in the blood.[39] With many people covering the skin to avoid sunburn and skin cancer, it may be that vitamin D levels are affected. The prevalence of vitamin D depletion in adults is believed to be increasing.[40]

Some countries produce fortified milk, which can boost the body's supply, and other sources include herring, mackerel, salmon, sardines, and cod- and halibut-liver oils. After the age of 70, the skin does not convert vitamin D as effectively, so dietary sources become even more important. Some experts recommend that women and men who don't get sun exposure and who eat less than four servings a day of fortified food could take a daily multiple vitamin which contains 400 I.U. (International Units) of vitamin D.

Magnesium

Magnesium's role in bone health appears to be significant. Magnesium influences bone metabolism and is also important for calcium regulation. (Although the optimum ratio of calcium to magnesium is not established, there is evidence that two parts calcium to one part magnesium will allow for better calcium absorption. Milk apparently has four parts calcium to one part magnesium.[41]) As much as 50 percent of the magnesium in the body is found in the bones.

Many researchers are now reporting that magnesium deficiency is common, and that it plays a big part in the development of osteoporosis. A typical American diet contains about 250 milligrams of magnesium, while the U.S. Recommended Daily Allowance (RDA) of magnesium is 350 milligrams. Moreover, some researchers believe that the optimal daily intake of this mineral is more than 600 milligrams. Magnesium is found in many foods (see page 187).

If levels of magnesium become depleted, bone growth stops. A magnesium deficiency can also affect the production of the biologically active form of vitamin D, and thereby further promote osteoporosis. A 1995 review on the role of magnesium states: "There is growing evidence that magnesium may be an important factor in the qualitative changes of the bone matrix that determine bone fragility."[42] The authors of the report note that bone mineral with decreased magnesium content results in larger abnormally shaped bone crystals, which may be more brittle than smaller, normal crystals. They add: "Trabecular bone from osteoporotic women has a reduced magnesium content and larger bone crystal formation than controls."

Studies have shown that women with low bone density tend to have a lower intake of magnesium than normal, and also have lower levels of magnesium in their blood and their bones.[43] A trial in Israel showed that postmenopausal women with osteoporosis (low BMD) could stop further bone loss by supplementing with 250 to 750 milligrams per day of magnesium for two years.[44] Eight percent of the women experienced a significant increase in bone density. Untreated controls lost bone density. Another study in Czechoslovakia found that 65 percent of women who supplemented with 1,500 to 3,000 milligrams of magnesium lactate daily for two years were rid of their pain and stopped further development of deformities of the vertebrae.[45]

A 1998 Austrian study of magnesium supplementation in young males found indications that magnesium suppressed high bone turnover, which could be beneficial in reducing associated bone loss.[46] Another Australian study investigating how a mother's diet during pregnancy affected her children's BMD, found that spinal bone density was significantly higher with the highest maternal intake of phosphorus, magnesium, and potassium. BMD was lower with a high maternal fat intake. According to the researchers, total body BMD was significantly associated with magnesium only.[47]

Calcium Sources

The body needs calcium, preferably from food, as opposed to supplements. The optimal calcium intake is not known. The World Health Organization recommends 400 to 500 milligrams of calcium per day for adults. The United States RDA is higher, and has steadily increased over the years. Initially, 800 milligrams per day was recommended, perhaps partly due to other factors known to have caused calcium loss, such as the consumption of meat and salt, use of tobacco prod-

> *The best-absorbed calcium sources are green, leafy vegetables, legumes, and seeds.*

ucts, and physical inactivity. Current recommendations range from 1,200 to 1,500 milligrams of calcium per day.

The best-absorbed calcium sources are green, leafy vegetables, legumes, and seeds. They have several advantages that dairy products lack. Dairy contains animal protein, and has comparatively low levels of magnesium. Vegetables and legumes contain antioxidants, complex carbohydrates, fiber, and iron, and have little fat and no cholesterol.

The body also absorbs calcium more efficiently when it comes from vegetables rather than dairy products. For example, calcium absorption from milk is approximately 32 percent, while calcium absorption from broccoli, Brussels sprouts, mustard greens, turnip greens, and kale ranges from 40 percent to 64 percent.[48] Spinach is an exception. It contains a large amount of calcium, but in a form that is poorly absorbed due to the presence of oxalic acid. Beans (e.g., pinto beans, black-eyed peas, and navy beans) and bean products (such as tofu) are rich in calcium and vegetable protein. Seaweed contains high amounts of calcium, phosphorus, magnesium, boron, iron, iodine, and sodium. It also contain vitamins A, B_I, C, E, and is one of the few vegetarian sources of vitamin B_{12}. Calcium and magnesium content in common foods is listed in the table on the next page.

CALCIUM AND MAGNESIUM IN FOODS		
SOURCE	Calcium (mg)	Magnesium (mg)
Barley (I cup, cooked)	17	35
Beet greens (I cup, boiled)	164	98
Bok choy (I cup))	158	19
Broccoli (I cup, boiled)	72	37
Brown rice (I cup, cooked)	20	84
Brussels sprouts (I cup, cooked)	56	31
Butternut squash (I cup, boiled)	46	22
Chickpeas (I cup, cooked)	80	79
Collards (I cup, boiled)	226	32
Dates, dried (I cup)	57	62
Figs, dried (10 medium)	275	110
Green beans (I cup, boiled)	58	31
Kale (I cup, boiled)	94	23
Kidney beans (I cup, boiled)	50	80
Lentils (I cup, boiled)	38	71
Lima beans (I cup, boiled)	32	81
Molasses, blackstrap (I Tbsp.)	172	43
Mustard greens (I cup, boiled)	104	21
Navel orange (I medium)	52	13
Navy beans (I cup, boiled)	127	107
Oatmeal, instant (I packet)	163	42
Okra (I cup, boiled)	101	91
Pinto beans (I cup, boiled)	82	94
Rhubarb, frozen, cooked	348	29
Raisins (I cup)	71	48
Soybeans (I cup, boiled)	175	148
Tofu (1/4 block)	131	37
Turnip greens (I cup, boiled)	197	32
Vegetarian baked beans (I cup)	127	81
White beans (I cup, boiled)	191	134

Source: USDA Nutrient Database

Vitamin K

Bone contains significant amounts of vitamin K, and low levels of vitamin K have been found in the blood of those with osteoporosis and in postmenopausal women. Vitamin K is required for the production of osteocalcin, a protein that attracts calcium to bone tissue and facilitates beneficial calcium crystal formation. Vitamin K supplements have been shown to increase this process (known as carboxylation) in postmenopausal women, thereby reducing bone loss. In controlled trials, people with low bone density given large amounts of vitamin K (45 milligrams per day) showed an increase in bone density after six months, and decreased bone loss after one year. [49]

Studies link insufficient vitamin K intake to fracture. Research at Harvard University found that women who consumed less than 109 micrograms a day sustained 30 percent more hip fractures over a 10-year period.[50] In the Framingham Heart Study between 1988 and 1995, 888 elderly men and women consumed various levels of vitamin K. Those averaging 56 micrograms per day experienced more hip fractures by 1995 than those reporting the highest intake levels of 254 micrograms per day. Researchers stated that vitamin K activates at least three proteins involved in bone health.[51]

Broccoli is a great source of vitamin K, as are leafy greens, legumes, and soybean oil. Scientists have known for years that astronauts lose bone density rapidly in space. A report in 2000 found a lack of vitamin K in astronauts, which may directly contribute to the space-related bone loss.[52] Because intestinal bacteria make 90 percent of vitamin K, people who have had frequent or long-term antibiotic use are likely to have insufficient vitamin K. Vitamin K is fat-soluble, and can be malabsorbed by those with chronic malabsorption or gastrointestinal problems.

Manganese

Manganese is a trace mineral, which is required for bone mineralization and the formation of connective tissue in cartilage and bone. In a study of Belgian women with osteoporosis (low BMD), blood levels of manganese were 75 percent lower than those of women without osteoporosis.[53] Basketball player Bill Walton's repeated fractures ceased after he began taking manganese supplements. Manganese, however, is toxic in high doses. The RDA is between 15 milligrams and 20 milligrams. Excellent sources of manganese include pecans, peanuts, pineapple fruit and juice, oatmeal, beans (pinto, lima, navy), rice, spinach, sweet potato, and whole wheat bread.

Zinc

Zinc, along with vitamin A and vitamin C, is essential for the formation of collagen. It enhances the biochemical action of vitamin D. Zinc levels have been found to be low in elderly people with osteoporosis. In one study, men consuming only 10 milligrams of zinc per day had almost twice the risk of osteoporotic fractures compared with those with significantly more zinc in their diets.[54] It has not yet been proven that zinc supplementation will prevent osteoporosis, but many doctors recommend that their patients supplement with 10-30 milligrams daily. Zinc is found in whole grain products, wheat bran and germ, brewer's yeast, and pumpkin seeds

Copper

Copper is needed for normal bone synthesis and is a factor in the strengthening of connective bone tissue. A placebo-controlled two-year study reported that 3 milligrams of copper daily prevented bone loss.[55] Although more research is required to confirm the role of copper in treating osteoporosis, many nutritionists recommend two to three milligrams per day, especially if the person is supplementing with zinc, as zinc will deplete copper levels. Copper is found naturally in liver, shellfish, leafy vegetables, legumes, grains, and spirulina. Water that is delivered through copper piping is also a good source.

Strontium

Strontium, the trace mineral (not to be confused with the radioactive substance of the same name), plays a crucial role in bone remodeling. It tends to migrate to sites in bone where active remodeling is taking place. Preliminary evidence suggests that women with fragility fractures may have reduced levels of this trace mineral. Several small studies have observed decreased bone pain, and an increase in bone formation in people taking quite high doses of strontium.[56] Most experts recommend between 1 and 3 milligrams per day. Strontium Ranelate, a new drug, appears to reduce the incidence of vertebral fractures in postmenopausal women with low bone density.

Boron

Boron, a trace element, appears to play an important role in bone building and strength. It has a role in parathyroid metabolism and influences the functions of calcium, magnesium, vitamin D, and phosphorus. Supplementation has been shown to increase the level of estrogen in some women. In a 1987 study, women taking 3 milligrams of supplemental boron for seven weeks lost 44 percent less calcium and 33 percent less magnesium in their urine than those not taking boron.[57] Boron deficiency has also been linked to arthritis, and there are indications that supplemental boron may provide relief. In areas where soil levels of boron are high, it has been noted that arthritis incidence is lower.[58]

Boron is safe when taken at the recommended daily dosage of 2 to 6 milligrams. It is found in sea vegetables, leafy vegetables, avocados, legumes, and nuts. Wine has also been shown to contain appreciable amounts of boron.

Silicon

Silicon is important for skin, hair, and in the formation of connective tissue, bone, and cartilage. The trace mineral combines with calcium and is highly concentrated at sites of growing bones. In preliminary research, supplementation with silicon increased bone mineral density in a group of eight women with low bone density.[59] Silica is found in hard, unprocessed grains and vegetables, especially cabbage, parsnips, asparagus, olives, and radishes. Horsetail and oatstraw teas are excellent sources of silica.

Betain

Individuals with osteoporosis often absorb calcium poorly. Low stomach acid (hypochlorhydria) is relatively common in women over the age of 50, and may reduce absorption of most forms of calcium. Betain is an acidifying agent for the entire gastrointestinal system that increases the absorption of bone building nutrients. It is found in specific supplements.

Folic Acid, Vitamin B_6, Vitamin B_{12}

These three are known to reduce levels of the amino acid homocysteine in the body. Homocystinuria, a condition associated with high homocysteine levels, is known to cause osteoporosis. Although no research exists on the effects of supplementation, normal amounts found in high-potency B-complex supplements should be adequate.[60] Pyroxidine (vitamin B_6) is required for collagen linking and the strength of connective bone tissue.

Folate (the form of folic acid found in foods) can be added to the diet through green, leafy vegetables, beans, and citrus fruits. Whole grain cereals, green cruciferous vegetables, lean meats and chicken, and dairy foods are good sources of vitamin B_6 and B_{12}.

Vitamin A & Vitamin C

Your body uses these to make collagen, which keeps bones flexible and strong. Animal studies have shown that osteoporosis can result from vitamin C deficiency.[61]

Too much vitamin A, however, can be harmful. High serum levels of retinol (Vitamin A) are associated with an increased risk for hip fracture in men, suggesting that the popularity of foods fortified with vitamin A may need to be reviewed.[62] Earlier studies suggest that vitamin A may prevent the formation of new bone and increase the risk of fractures. A Swedish study examined 247 women with hip fracture as compared with 873 women in a control group. Researchers found that, for every 1 milligram-per-day (3,333 I.U.) increase in vitamin A (retinol), the risk of hip fracture increased by 68 percent. While it is essential for the formation of collagen, excessive dietary intake of vitamin A appears to be linked to an increased risk for hip fracture.[63] Most fruits have high vitamin C content – especially citrus fruits, berries, apples, pineapples, and tomatoes.

Vitamin E

It is known that free radical activity may increase bone resorption. A preliminary report on the effectiveness of vitamin E in preventing bone loss in animals suggests that supplementation may be a way to reverse free-radical damage in bone.[64] Good sources of vitamin E include wheat germ, sunflower seeds, pine nuts, sun-dried tomatoes, and almonds.

Essential Fatty Acids

Supplementing with fish oil may improve calcium metabolism in older women with osteoporosis. A preliminary study examined older women of average age 80 with osteoporosis (low BMD) who took 4 grams of fish oil (gamma-linolenic acid) every day for four months. Researchers found that the women had higher blood levels of calcium, improved calcium absorption, and chemicals in their urine indicating bone formation. When fish oil was combined with evening primrose oil (gamma-linoleic acid), there was an increase in bone density of 3.1 percent over a three-year period.[65] This is a significant outcome in older women, and more research is needed in this important area.

Bone Care Nutrients

A well-balanced diet provides the best source of nutrients. If your diet is inadequate, or you wish to make sure you are getting the essentials, you might consider a mineral and vitamin supplement. Consult your health-care provider to help ascertain which supplement is best for you. Be aware that certain vitamin and mineral supplements can interact with medications.

Summary

Research indicates that dietary and lifestyle choices influence bone strength and health. A fundamental prevention and treatment strategy includes a diet that emphasizes the consumption of fresh vegetables, leafy greens, vegetable proteins, and avoids refined foods, heavy meats, caffeine, and carbonated drinks. The adequate intake of essential bone nutrients is also essential. These approaches will benefit overall health, as well as bone health. Indeed, embracing a healthy diet, receiving recommended amounts of vitamins and minerals, and adhering to a regular exercise program may be the most effective means to prevent bone loss and fragility fracture.

✳ I I ✳

A Family Story,
10 Years Later

Living with low bone density.

In just two decades, osteoporosis has gone from being a rare bone disease to being a major health threat. The World Health Organization predicts a global epidemic of osteoporosis by 2050, and the National Osteoporosis Foundation warns of fragility fractures occurring every 20 seconds in the United States. A proliferation of glossy advertisements encourages fearful mid-life women to adopt bone density screening and bone-sparing drugs to avert debilitating hip fracture and painful curvature of the spine. The message has been so compelling it is not surprising that physicians and their patients have universally accepted it.

While medicine, at its core, is about preventing and healing illness, medicine is also about big business — billions of dollars annually.

Giant public relations machines promote treatments and cures, but they increasingly promote diseases and epidemics as well. Marketing campaigns often capitalize on people's fears of aging and illness. Osteoporosis exemplifies this. It has become one of the most commercially profitable diseases ever because it diagnoses and treats the well. Women and men throughout the world have been convinced that by virtue of normal, age-related bone loss, they are at risk for a serious disease.

It simply isn't true.

Here are the facts:

- Loss of bone density is a normal aspect of growing older and is a condition that may never manifest as disease.

- Most people who have low bone density will not fracture, and the majority of fractures occur in people who *do not* have osteoporosis (low BMD).

- Hip fractures — the real fear surrounding osteoporosis — result from many contributing factors. Preventing falls in the elderly will decrease hip fractures far more effectively than drugs to treat low bone density.

- Most osteoporosis drugs do not help the majority of people taking them and in some cases may exacerbate a patient's condition. They can carry risks that may surface years later

- The best bone-strengthening treatments come from lifestyle choices each individual has control over: eating nutritious foods, getting regular exercise, lowering exposure to chemical toxins, and managing stress.

Modern medicine is an essential part of our lives. The vast majority of medical practitioners are compassionate caregivers who act sincerely in the best interests of their patients, and many people suffering acute and serious diseases benefit greatly from medical intervention. However, medical intervention, specifically drug treatment, must be administered on the basis of sound research and study – and with careful assessment of the benefits and risks. The risks cannot be understated. Prescription drugs cause more than 106,000 deaths annually in the United States.

Physicians bear a tremendous responsibility in administering care, and patients bear an equally large responsibility – their own health. We must cultivate a healthy, open-minded skepticism and willingness to question diagnoses, while educating ourselves about the safety and effectiveness of any treatment before embarking on it. By challenging and questioning current practices, we can contribute to creating greater rigor in science and better health care for all.

Living with Low Bone Density

There is no doubt that osteoporosis, characterized by fragility fractures, is a disease with potentially serious consequences. Established osteoporosis, however, is a rare disease linked to many factors. Osteoporosis, defined by low bone density alone, is a condition that most of us can live with and suffer no ill effects.

Eleven members of my family spanning three generations have a diagnosis of either osteoporosis or osteopenia. It is almost 10 years since we were diagnosed, and although it is clear there is a genetic factor involved, there is still virtually nothing known about the condition. It is labeled "idiopathic" — of unknown cause. In this sense it differs from age-related osteoporosis as discussed in this book. It is interesting to observe however, that in all this time, none of us has fractured. Neither has the diagnosis limited our ability to enjoy life.

My daughter, Camille, was only 16 when she was told that she had the bones of an 80-year-old. In typical teenage style, she didn't discuss it much. Her father and I had little information on the disease and were very worried. Camille appeared to be getting on with her life, but years later told me that the diagnosis had affected her tremendously. She feared more painful fractures and cut back on physical activity, believing her fragile bones could not withstand any knocks or pressure. She avoided sports at school and no longer went skiing. She even gave up dancing, which was especially hard, as she had been passionate about it from an early age. All of this was quite the opposite of what she ought to have done — but no such advice was given.

As time went by and she continued to be fracture-free, Camille's confidence returned. At 18, she graduated from high school in New Zealand and set off on a working holiday, backpacking through Asia and Europe. Over the next two years, she explored the islands of Indonesia, climbed the High Atlas Mountains in Morocco, worked in a London sushi restaurant, and traveled through Europe, India, and Nepal. She settled for some time in Japan, before returning to New Zealand to train as a graphic designer. These days she is physically active and fit; she lifts weights and exercises regularly. She is passionate about dancing and is a member of a modern dance troupe that performs vigorous, high-impact floor routines that fragile bones would not tolerate. Camille has sustained no fractures for almost 10 years.

My parents are fit and active, and both enjoy very good health. Their story has been told in a previous chapter. My brother Geoff has "severe" osteopenia. He farms a large block of land, and his lifestyle demands constant physical activity. He is extremely fit and enjoys competition tennis, badminton, skiing, and surfboarding. In 1988, he suffered multiple broken bones when his tractor rolled on him. He is lucky to have survived. These high-impact fractures, obviously, cannot be linked to osteoporosis. Testament to his good health, he made a complete recovery and remains fracture-free today. He tells me that he doesn't give a thought about his diagnosis of low bone density.

My son, Jude, has very low bone density, enough to qualify him for a diagnosis of osteoporosis. Although he fractured his wrist in a heavy fall from gymnastics equipment at age 14 and twice broke a finger while playing basketball, he has remained fracture-free for 15 years. He lives with his wife in Canada and has continued to be active, enjoying mountain biking, skiing, and in-line skating. He maintains that the diagnosis has not affected his life in any way.

My husband, Stewart, has bone density considerably lower than the threshold for osteoporosis, putting him in an "extreme risk" category. Yet, other than a minor crack in a wrist bone as a child, he has never fractured. He was very athletic when young, playing competition rugby and winning high-jump awards. He is a strong, healthy, physically active person who doesn't fit the image of a fragile person. He is a home handyman who balks at nothing — lifting heavy objects, climbing high trees to prune them, painting the roof, building fences, sheds, and furniture, gardening, and laying concrete and wooden floors. Interestingly, until I reminded him of his diagnosis, he had forgotten how supposedly serious it was. He was momentarily alarmed before shrugging his shoulders and dismissing it. He figures that by continuing to take care of his physical, mental, and spiritual health, he is doing the best that he can to avert future problems. Because so much is not known about osteoporosis, chances are that his bones are strong and flexible, and the low BMD reading is meaningless.

My last DXA scan indicated that I had "serious osteopenia," meaning low bone density, but not in the osteoporosis category. I had four nonserious wrist fractures as a child, but haven't had any others since age 14.

I come from a family of gardeners. Gardening is great weight-bearing exercise that enhances flexibility and improves muscle and bone strength. My grandfather who lost a leg in the World War I was still digging his prolific garden when he was 90. My sister Julie and her husband, David, have a two-and-a-half-acre garden that they have single-handedly established over 28 years. They have woodlands, weeping pear trees, delicate maples, and primulas grown from seed collected in China. There are massive oaks, established borders, native trees and grasses, and rare, exquisite alpine blooms. They have a huge vegetable garden and produce abundant organic vegetables and fruit year-round. They are adventurers too, and in recent years they have traveled the Karakoram Highway through the Hindu Kush Mountains from China to Pakistan; climbed the lower reaches of the Tibetan plateau on a botanical pilgrimage; survived high altitudes traveling in Tibet; and taken a boat down the mighty Mekong river in Laos, negotiating its waterways and canals where it reaches the ocean in Vietnam. Julie has osteopenia too, but she has never fractured. She is now 53 and is very fit. In addition to working full time as a librarian, she skis, hikes, and walks on the beach every morning.

My sister Barbara is now 56 and has severe osteoporosis. She has been advised that she is at high risk of fracture and must take long-term bisphosphonate treatment. She is the head of the school of languages at a local polytechnic school. Her children are grown, and she and her husband have taken to traveling again to places like Egypt, Cambodia, and Europe. They have a beautiful, rural property and work their garden, growing trees, organic vegetables, and fruit. Every morning Barbara walks the hills and tracks beside the sea through the native trees that circle their land. She loves her patch of coastal New Zealand and the deep connection she has with it. She eats well, making sure that her diet includes lots of fresh vegetables, nuts, seeds, grains, and essential fatty acids. She has not had a fracture since she was 7 years old.

I do not dismiss the potential for problems for my son, daughter, and other family members later in life. Our history of childhood fracture and the very low bone density in some of us could increase our risk for fragility fracture. A dire prognosis, however, is far from confirmed: A wide biological variation in bone density exists among healthy adults; perhaps our low bone density is normal for us, and our bone strength and micro-architecture is sound. As medical science continues to grapple with understanding bone health over the course of a person's lifetime, no one can say what the future holds.

In setting out to learn all I could about osteoporosis I have uncovered myth and misinformation every step of the way. Thankfully, the status quo can change There is now debate in the medical community over the appropriateness of testing and treating well women for a disease that they may never have; and there are ongoing questions about the accuracy of diagnosis and about the safety and effectiveness of treatments.

My research has confirmed that we must each take responsibility for our well-being and for making wise choices. I believe this book to be optimistic and reassuring. I hope that it gives women the courage to deeply question their physicians, and that it encourages them to continue on their own journey of education and self-discovery. Menopause is not a disease; neither is growing old. These are rewarding years when we can take positive action to assure long and healthy lives.

Notes

CHAPTER 2: The Myth of Risk

[1]Ahmed, A.I.H. et al. "Screening for osteopenia and osteoporosis: do the accepted normal ranges lead to overdiagnosis?" *Osteoporosis International* 1997;7:432-438.

[2]Rubin, S.M., Cummings, S.R. "Results of bone densitometry affect women's decisions about takng measures to prevent fractures." *Annals of Internal Medicine* 1992;116(12 Pt.1):990-5.

[3]Marci, C.D, Viechnicki, M.B., Greenspan, S.L. "Bone mineral densitometry substantially influences health-related behaviors of postmenopausal women." *Calcified Tissue International.* 2000 Feb;66(2):113-118.

[4]Pors Nielson, S. "The fallacy of BMD: a critical review of the diagnostic use of dual X-ray absorptiometry." *Clinical Rheumatology* 2000;19(3):174-183.

[5]Heaney, R.P. "Sources of bone fragility." *Osteoporosis International* 2000;Suppl.2:S43-46.

[6]Weinsier, R.L. "Dairy foods and bone health: Examination of the evidence." *American Journal of Clinical Nutrition* 2000;72:681-9.

[7]Lopez, J.M. et al. "Bone turnover and density in healthy women during breastfeeding and after weaning." *Osteoporosis International* 1996;6:153-59.

[8]National Osteoporosis Foundation (U.S.) Web site: http://www.nof.org/

[9]http://www.nof.org/news/pressreleases/prevmo_2001.html

[10]Lau, E.M.C. "The epidemiology of hip fracture in Asia: An update." *Osteoporosis International* 1996 Suppl.3:S19-S23.

[11]International Osteoporosis Foundation Web site: http://www.osteofound.org/press_centre/scrip_magazine.html

[12]Dequeker, J. et al. "Hip fracture and osteoporosis in a XIIth Dynasty female skeleton from Lisht, Upper Egypt." *Journal of Bone and Mineral Research* 1997;12(6):881-888.

[13]Green, C.J., Bassett, K., Foerster, V., Kazanjian, A. "Bone Mineral Testing: Does the evidence support its selective use in well women?" British Columbia Office of Health Technology Assessment. Dec 1997. www.chspr.ubc.ca

[14]http://washingtonpost.com/wp-dyn/articles/A14106-2000Sep25.html

[15]Kazanjian, A., Green, C., Bassett, K. "Normal bone mass, aging bodies, marketing of fear: Bone mineral density screening of well women." British Columbia Office of Health Technology Assessment. Sept 1998. www.chspr.ubc.ca

[16]Green, C.J., Bassett, K., Foerster, V., Kazanjian, A. Ibid.

[17]Ott, Susan, M.D., "Osteoporosis and bone physiology." Web site: http://courses.washington.edu/bonephys/opclin.html

[18]Genant, H.K. et al. "Interim report and recommendations of the WHO Task-Force for Osteoporosis." *Osteoporosis International* 1999;19:259-264.

[19]Ott, Susan, M.D. Correspondence with the author. April 3, 2001.

[20]Keating, N.L. et al. "Use of hormone replacement by postmenopausal women in the United States." *Annals of Internal Medicine* 1999;130(7):545-53.

[21]Women's Health Initiative HRT Update 2001. http://www.nhlbi.nih.gov/whi/

[22]Writing Group for the Women's Health Initiative Investigators. "Risks and benefits of estrogen plus progestin in healthy postmenopausal women." *Journal of the American Medical Association* 2002;288:321-333.

[23]WHO Geneva 1994. "Assessment of fracture risk and its application to screening for postmenopausal osteoporosis." WHO technical report series 843.

[24]Ringertz, H. et al. "Bone density measurement: a systematic review. A report from SBU, the Swedish Council on Technology Assessment in Health Care." *Journal of Internal Medicine* 1997;241(Suppl. 739):i-iii, 1-60.

[25]Dewar, Elaine. "Breaking news: blowing the whistle on osteoporosis." *Homemakers*, October 1998; 57- 70.

[26]Davis, J.W. et al. "The peak bone mass of Hawaiian, Filipino, Japanese, and white women living in Hawaii." *Calcified Tissue International* 1994;55:249-52.

[27]Melton, L.J. III et al. "Effects of body size and skeletal site on the estimated prevalence of osteoporosis in women and men." *Osteoporosis International* 2000:11:977-983.

[28]Green, C.J., Bassett K., Foerster V., Kazanjian A. Ibid.

[29]Pors Neilsen, S. Ibid.

[30]Polner, F. "Osteoporosis: Looking at the whole picture." *Medical World News* 1985;14 Jan:38-58. Cited in Coney, S. *The Menopause Industry*. Penguin Books NZ. 1992. p.107.

[31]Law, M.R. et al. "Strategies for prevention of osteoporosis and hip fracture." *British Medical Journal* 1991;303: 453-459.

[32]Coney S. Ibid.

[33]Ott, Susan, M.D., "Osteoporosis and bone physiology". http://courses.washington.edu/bonephys/

[34]http://www.nof.org/

[35]Tenenhouse, A. et al. "Estimation of the prevalence of low bone density in Canadian women and men using a population-specific DXA reference standard: The Canadian Multicentre Osteoporosis Study (CaMos)." *Osteoporosis International* 2000;11:897-904.

[36]Looker, A.C. et al. "Prevalence of low femoral density in older US women. National Health and Nutrition Examination Survey III (NHANES III)." *Journal of Bone and Mineral Research* 1995;10:796-802.

[37]http://www.osteofound.org/

[38]www.nos.org.uk

[39]http://www.osteofound.org/member_societies/australia2.html

[40]http://osteoporosis.org.nz/links.html

[41]NZ Herald. Monday, April 23, 2001.

[42]Ott, Susan M.D. Correspondence with the author. November 2000.

[43]Heaney, R. P. Ibid.

[44]Green, C.J., Bassett K., Foerster V., Kazanjian A. Ibid.

[45]Kazanjian, A. et al. "BMD testing in social context." *International Journal of Technology Assessment in Health Care* 1999;15 (4):679-685.

[46]Green, C.J., Bassett K., Foerster V., Kazanjian A. Ibid.

[47]Walker, A., "Osteoporosis and Calcium Deficiency," *American Journal of Clinical Nutrition* 1965; 16: 327 - 336.

[48]Starfield, Barbara. "Is US health really the best in the world?" *Journal of the American Medical Association* 2000; 284 (4):483-5.

CHAPTER 3: The Myth of Diagnosis

[1]Ott, Susan M.D., "Osteoporosis and bone physiology." http://courses.washington.edu/bonephys/opbmd.html#young

[2]Green, C.J., Bassett, K., Foerster, V., Kazanjian, A. "Bone Mineral Testing: Does the evidence support its selective use in well women?" B.C. Office of Health Technology Assessment. Dec 1997. ww.chspr.ubc.ca

[3]Genant, H.K. et al. "Interim report and recommendations of the WHO Task-Force for Osteoporosis." *Osteoporosis International* 1999;19:259-264

[4]Heaney, R.P. "Sources of Bone Fragility." *Osteoporosis International* 2000. Suppl 2:S43-46.

[5]Ott, Susan M.D. Correspondence with the author. November 2000.

[6]Ott, Susan M.D. Ibid.

[7]Karlsson, M.K. et al. "Bone mineral normative data in Malmo, Sweden; Comparison with reference data and hip fracture incidence in other ethnic groups." *Acta Orthopaedica Scandinavica* 1993;64(2):168-72 (Cited in BCHOTA Review. www.chspr.ubc.ca)

[8]Law, M.R. et al. "Strategies for prevention of osteoporosis and hip fracture." *British Medical Journal* 1991;303: 453-459.

[9]Ibid.

[10]Melton, L.J. III et al. "Effects of body size and skeletal site on the estimated prevalence of osteoporosis in women and men." *Osteoporosis International* 2000:11:977-983.

[11]Kanis, J.A. et al. "An update on the diagnosis and assessment of osteoporosis with densitometry." Position Paper. *Osteoporosis International* 2000;11:192-202.

[12]Pors Nielson, S. "The fallacy of BMD: a critical review of the diagnostic use of dual X-ray absorptiometry." *Clinical Rheumatology* 2000;19:174-183.

[13]Ibid.

[14]Miller, P.D. et al "Prediction of fracture risk in postmenopausal white women with peripheral bone densitometry: evidence from the National Osteoporosis Risk Assessment." *Journal of Bone and Mineral Research* 2002;17(12):222-30.

[15]Dewar, Elaine. "Breaking news: blowing the whistle on the osteoporosis epidemic." *Homemaker's* 1998 October 1998;57- 70.

[16]Law, M.R. et al. Ibid.

[17]Bachrach, L.K. "Acquisition of optimal bone mass in childhood and adolescence." *Trends in Endocrinology and Metabolism* January-February 2001;12(1):22-8.

[18]Ibid.

[19]Kanis, J.A. et al Ibid.

[20]Green, C.J., Bassett, K., Foerster, V., Kazanjian, A. Ibid.

[21]Looker, A.C. et al. "Prevalence of low femoral bone density in older US women from NHANES III." *Journal of Bone and Mineral Research* 1995: (10) 5:796-802.

[22]Kanis, J.A. et al Ibid.

[23]Tenenhouse, A., et al. "Estimation of the prevalence of low bone density in Canadian women and men using a population-specific DXA reference standard: The Canadian Multicentre Osteoporosis Study (CaMos)." *Osteoporosis International* 2000; 11:897-904.

[24]Gurlek, A. et al. "Inappropriate reference range for peak bone mineral density in dual-energy X-ray absorptiometry: Implications for the interpretation of T-scores." *Osteoporosis International* 2000; 11; 9: 809- 813.

[25]Ibid.

[26]Ahmed, A. I. H., et al. "Screening for osteopenia and osteoporosis: Do the accepted normal ranges lead to overdiagnosis?" *Osteoporosis International* 1997:7:432-438.

[27]Simmons, A. et al. "Dual energy X-ray absorptiometry normal reference range use within the UK and the effect of different normal ranges on the assessment of bone density." *British Journal of Radiology* 1995;68(812):903-9.

[28]Ahmed, A. I. H., et al. Ibid.

[29]Pors Nielsen S. Ibid.

[30]Delmas, P.D. "Do we need to change the WHO definition of osteoporosis?" *Osteoporosis International* 2000;11:189-191.

[31]Green, C.J., Bassett, K., Foerster, V., Kazanjian, A. Ibid.

[32]Kazanjian, A. et al. "BMD testing in social context." *International Journal of Technology Assessment in Health Care* 1999;15:679-685.

[33]Marci, C..D. et al. "Bone mineral densitometry substantially influences health-related behaviors of postmenopausal women." *Calcified Tissue International* 2000 Feb;66(2):113-118.

[34]Varney, L.F. et al. "Classification of osteoporosis and osteopenia in postmenopausal women is dependent on site-specific analysis." *Journal of Clinical Densitometry* 1999;2:275-83.

[35]Varney, L.F. et al. Ibid .

[36]Green, C.J., Bassett, K., Foerster, V., Kazanjian, A. Ibid.

[37]Homick, J. Bailey, D. "Bone density measurement: a health technology report." 1999 Alberta Heritage Foundation for Medical Research.

[38]Cited in BCOHTA review: www.chspr.ubc.ca

[40]Ibid.

[41]Hailey, D. et al. "INAHTA Project on the effectiveness of density measurement and associated treatments for prevention of fractures." Statement of findings. September 1996. http://www.ahfmr.ab.ca/hta/hta-publications/joint/bdm.stmt.shtml

[42]Ibid.

[43]Bassett, K. "On trying to stop the measurement of bone density to sell drugs: A tribute to a friend." *Tales from Other Drug Wars.* Papers from the 12th Annual Health policy Conference, held in Vancouver, B.C., Nov. 26, 1999. ISBN 0-88865-240-2

[44]Ibid.

[45]Green, C.J., Bassett, K., Foerster, V., Kazanjian, A. Ibid.

[46]Heaney, R.P. et al. "Peak bone mass." *Osteoporosis International* 2000;11:985-1009.

[47]Ibid.

[48]Dewar Elaine. Ibid.

[49]Homick J., Bailey D. Ibid.

[50]Effectiveness Bulletin from the University of Leeds. A Review: Bandolier evidence-based health care. http://www.jr2.ox.ac.uk/bandolier/band3/b3-4.html

CHAPTER 4: The Myth of Causality

[1]Cited in "Osteoporosis and bone physiology." The Web site of Susan Ott, M.D., Associate Professor of Medicine at the University of Washington. http://courses.washington.edu/bonephys/

[2]Osteoporosis Prevention, Diagnosis, and Therapy. US National Institute of Health (NIH) Consensus Statement March 2000.

[3]Ibid.

[4]http://courses.washington.edu/bonephys/opdem.html

[5]Hayes, W.C. et al. "Etiology and prevention of age-related hip fractures." *Bone* 1996;18:77S-86S.

[6]Ott, Susan M.D. Personal correspondence, Oct. 16, 2000.

[7]U.S. National Institute of Health (NIH) Consensus Statement, March 2000. Ibid.

[8]McGrother, C.W. et al, "Evaluation of a hip fracture risk score for assessing elderly women: The Melton Osteoporotic Fracture (MOF) Study." *Osteoporosis International* 2002; 13: 89-96.

[9]http://courses.washington.edu/bonephys/opclin.html

[10]Holmes, J. et al. "Psychiatric assessment advised for patients with hip fracture." *Lancet* 2001;357:1264.

[11]Mautalen, C.A .et al. "Are the etiologies of cervical and trochanteric hip fractures different?" *Bone* 1996;18:133S-137S.

[12]Cummings, S.R. et al. "Racial differences in hip axis length might explain racial differences in rates of hip fracture." *Osteoporosis International* 1994; 4: 226-229.

[13]Homick. J., Bailey, D. "Bone density measurement: a health technology report." Alberta Heritage Foundation for Medical Research. http:/www.ahfmr.ab.ca/hta

[14]Cummings, S.R. et al. "Risk factors for hip fracture in white women." *New England Journal of Medicine.* 1995;332(12)767-73.

[15]Ibid.

[16]Cumming, R. G., Klineberg, R. J., *American Journal of Epidemiology* 1994; 139: 493-503.

[17]Report on the International Osteoporosis Foundation World Congress on Osteoporosis, Lisbon Portugal 2002. www.medscape.com/viewprogam/1889

[18]"Padded clothing prevents life-threatening hip fractures." *Advance for Physical Therapists and PT Assistants* Nov. 2, 2000.

[19]Cryer, C., et al. "Hip protector compliance among older people living in residential care homes." *Injury Prevention* 2002: 8, 202-206.

[20]Wallace, R. "Hip pads to prevent fractures in older people." *National Institute of Nursing Research* http://www.nih.gov/ninr/news-info/resdirections/hippads.html

[21]Ott, Susan. M.D., Ibid. Web site: http://courses.washington.edu/bonephys/

[22]Heaney, R. P. "Bone mass, fragility and the decision to treat." (Editorial). *JAMA* 1998;280;24:2119-2120.

[23]Frost, H.M. "Personal experience in managing acute compression fractures, their aftermath, and the bone pain syndrome in osteoporosis." *Osteoporosis International* 1998;8:13-15.

[24]Bennell, K. et al. "The role of physiotherapy in the prevention and treatment of osteoporosis." *Manual Therapy* 2000;5(4):198-213.

[25]Doherty, D. et al. "Lifetime and five-year age-specific risks of first and subsequent osteoporotic fractures in postmenopausal women." *Osteoporosis International* 2001;12: 16-23.

[26]Ott, Susan M.D. Correspondence with the author, 2001.

[27]Lunt,M. et al. "Population-Based geographic variations in DXA bone density in Europe: The EVOS study." *Osteoporosis International* 1997;7:175-189.

[28]Ettinger, B. Email correspondence with the author. Apr 23, 2001.

[29]http://www.studd.co.uk/osteoporosis.html

[30]http://courses.washington.edu/bonephys/

[31]Pors Neilsen, S. "The fallacy of BMD: A critical review of the diagnostic use of dual X-ray absorptiometry." *Clinical Rheumatology* 2000. 19:174-183.

[32]Myers, E.R. et al. "Geometric variables from DXA of the radius predict forearm fracture load in vitro." *Calcified Tissue International* 1993;52:199-204.

[33]Osteoporosis Prevention, Diagnosis, and Therapy. NIH Consensus Statement 2000 March 27-29; 17(1): 1-36.

[34]Ibid.

[35]Ibid.

[36]Ibid.

[37]Orwoll, E.S. "Determinants of bone mineral density in older men." *Osteoporosis International* 2000;11:815-821.

[38]Ibid.

[39]Ibid.

[40]"Corticosteroid treatment increased risk of vertebral fracture." Presented at the meeting of the American Society for Bone and Mineral Research and the International Bone and Mineral Society. San Francisco Dec. 14, 1998.

[41]Tannirandorn P., Epstein S. Ibid.

[42]Ibid.

[43]Ibid.

[44]Ibid.

[45]Tannirandorn P., Epstein S. Ibid.

[46]Robinson, E. "Use of hormone replacement therapy to reduce the risk of osteopenia in adolescent girls with anorexia nervosa." *Journal of Adolescent Health* 2000 May;26(5):343-8.

[47]Ibid.

[48]Fasano, A. et al "Prevalence of celiac disease in at-risk and not-at-risk groups in the United States. A large multicenter study." *Archives of Internal Medicine*. 2003;163:286-292.

[49]Sategna-Guidetti, C., et al. "The effectsof 1-year gluten withdrawal on bone mass, bone metabolsim and nutritional status in newly-diagnosed adult coeliac disease patients." *Alimentary Pharmacology and Therapeutics* 2000 Jan:14(1):35-43.

CHAPTER 5: Overview of Drug Treatments

[1]Women's Health Initiative 2001 HRT Update. Participants' Web site http://www.whi.org/update/2001update.asp

[2]Fletcher, S.W. and Colditz, G.A. "Failure of estrogen plus progestin therapy for prevention." *Journal of the American Medical Association* 2002;288:366-368.

[3]Fugh-Berman, A., Pearson, C. "The over-selling of hormone replacement therapy." *Pharmacotherapy* 2002; 22(9):1295 -1208.

[4]Writing group for the Women's Health Initiative Investigators. "Risks and benefits of estrogen plus progestin in healthy postmenopausal women." *Journal of the American Medical Association* 2002;288:321-333.

[5]Grady, Deborah. "Hormone Replacement Therapy" (Real Audio file). Talk of the Nation radio interview, Friday, July 26, 2002   http://www.womens-health.org.nz/hrt.htm#radio

[6]National Institutes of Health News Release. July 9, 2002. www.nhlbi.nih.gov/new/press/02-07-09.htm

[7]Fletcher, S.W. , Colditz, G.A. Ibid.

[8]Fugh-Berman, A., Pearson, C. Ibid.

[9]Hulley, S., Grady, D., Bush, T. et al. "Randomized trial of estrogen plus progestin for secondary prevention of heart disease in postmenopausal women." *Journal of the American Medical Association.* 1998;280:605-641.

[10]Grady,D. , Cummings, S.R. "Postmenopausal hormone replacement therapy for prevention of fractures. How good is the evidence?" *Journal of the American Medical Association* 2001;285(22)2090-2100.

[11]Nelson, H., Humphrey, L., LeBlanc E. et al. "Postmenopausal hormone replacement therapy for the primary prevention of chronic conditions: a summary of the evidence for the U.S. Preventive Services Task Force." Available at: http://www.ahrq.gov/clinic/3rduspstf/hrt/hrtsum1.htm. Accessed: 11/12/2002.

[12]Cummings, S.R, Browner, W.S., Bauer, D. et al. "Endogenous hormones and the risk of hip and vertebral fractures among older women." *New England Journal of Medicine* 1998; 339;733-738.

[13]Sellmann, S. "Osteoporosis – the Myths." *Nexus Magazine* 1998;5(6). http://www.nexusmagazine.com/Osteoporosis.html

[14]Riggs, B., Melton, L. "Involutional Osteoporosis." *New England Journal of Medicine* 1986 26:1676-86.

[15]Heaney, R. "Bone mass, bone fragility and the decision to treat." *Journal of the American Medical Association* 1998;280(24):2119-2120.

[16]Riggs, L.B., Hodgson, S.F., O'Fallon, M . et al. " Effect of fluoride treatment on the fracture rate of postmenopausal women with osteoporosis." *New England Journal of Medicine* 1990;322:802-809.

[17]Cummings, S.R, et al. "Effect of Alendronate on risk of fracture in women with low bone density but without vertebral fractures." *Journal of the American Medical Association* 1998;280 (24):1077-2082.

[18]Therapeutics Letter, issue 20, July - August 1997 http://www.interchg.ubc.ca/jauca/pages/letter20.htm#alendronate

[19]Black, D.M., Cummings, S.R. et al. "Randomised trial of effect of alendronate on risk of fracture in women with existing vertebral fractures." *Lancet* 1996;348:1535-41.

[20]Cummings, S.R. et al. Ibid.

[21]Harris, S.T. "New considerations in the selection of current therapies to prevent and treat osteoporosis." CME Medscape December 2002. www.medscape.com/viewprogram/2185

[22]Seeman, E. "Treatment of asymptomatic osteopenic menopausal women." *Medscape Ob/Gyn & Women's Health* 2002. Available at: http://www.medscape.com/viewarticle/446109?mpid=7785

[23]Seeman, E. "Understanding how antiresorptive agents optimize therapeutic effect." *Medscape* 2002 Available at; http://www.medscape.com/viewarticle/443214

[24]Grady, D. "Hormone Replacement Therapy." Talk of the Nation radio interview. Friday, July 26, 2002 (Real Audio file). Available at the Web site: http://www.womens-health.org.nz/hrt.htm#radio

[25]Kavanagh, A.M. et al. "Hormone replacement therapy and accuracy of mammographic screening." *Lancet* 2000;355:270-4.

[26]Smith, W.A. et al. "Alcohol and breast cancer in women: a pooled analysis of cohort studies." Department of Nutrition, Harvard School of Public Health, Boston, Mass. *Journal of the American Medical Association* 1998 Feb, 279:7, 535-40.

[27]Lacey, J.V. et al. "Menopausal hormone replacement therapy and risk of ovarian cancer." *Journal of the American Medical Association* 2002;228:334-341.

[28]New Zealand Guidelines Group. "The appropriate prescribing of hormone replacement therapy." May 2001. www.nzgg.org.nz

[29]Hulley, S. et al. "Randomized trial of estrogen plus progestin for secondary prevention of coronary heart disease in postmenopausal women." *Journal of the American Medical Association* 1998;280:695-613.

[30]Kerr, M. "Combination hormone therapy increases women's stroke risk, even in first year." *Reuters Health* Feb 14, 2003.

[31]Grodstein, F. et al. "A prospective observational study of postmenopausal hormone therapy and primary prevention of cardiovascular disease." *Annals of Internal Medicine* 2000;133:933-941.

[32]Writing group for the Women's Health Initiative Investigators. "Risks and benefits of estrogen plus progestin in healthy postmenopausal women." *Journal of the American Medical Association* 2002;288:321-333.

[33]Grodstein, F. et al. "Postmenopausal hormone use and cholecystectomy in a large prospective study." *Obstetrics and Gynecology* 1994;83(1):5-11.

[34]Meier, C.R. et al. "Postmenopausal estrogen replacement therapy and the risk of developing lupus erythematosus or discoid lupus." *Journal of Rheumatology* 1998;25(8):1515-9.

[35]New Zealand Guidelines Group. Ibid.

[36]Barr, G. R. Harvard Medical School. Reporting to the American College of Chest Physicians. Oct. 26, 2000.

CHAPTER 6: The Myth of Safety

[1]Mashiba, T. et al. "Suppressed bone turnover by bisphosphonates increases microdamage accumulation and reduces some biomechanical properties in dog rib." *Journal of Bone and Mineral Research* 2000;15:613-620.

[2]Seeman, E.. "Understanding how antiresorptive agents optimize therapeutic effect." Medscape 2002Available at; http://www.medscape.com/viewarticle/443214

[3]Ott, Susan, M.D. Correspondence with the author, November 22, 2000.

[4]Ott, Susan, M.D. Web site: http://courses.washington.edu/bonephys/

[5]Kaunitz, A.M. "Osteopenia in a Premenopausal Woman." *Medscape Ob/Gyn & Women's Health* 8(1), 2003. Available at: http://www.medscape.com/viewarticle/447116

[6]Black, D.M. et al. "Randomised effect of alendronate on risk of fracture in women with existing vertebral fractures." *Lancet* 1996;348:1535-1541.

[7]Cummings, S.R. et al. "Effect of alendronate on risk of fracture in women with low bone density but without vertebral fractures." Results from The Fracture Intervention Trial. *Journal of the American Medical Association* 280;24:1998.

[8]Heaney, R.P. "Bone mass, bone fragility and the decision to treat." *Journal of the American Medical Association* 1998;280(24):2119-2120.

[9]Ettinger, B. et al. "Alendronate use among 812 women: prevalence of gastrointestinal complaints, noncompliance with patient instructions, and discontinuation." *Journal of Managed Care Pharmacy* 1998;4:488-492.

[10]Graham, D.Y. et al. "Alendronate and naproxen are synergistic for development of gastric ulcers." *Archives of Internal Medicine* 2001;161: 107-110.

[11]Harris, S.T. et al. "Effects of risedronate treatment on vertebral and non-vertebral fractures in women with postmenopausal osteoporosis: a randomized controlled trial." *Journal of the American Medical Association* 1999;282:1344-1352.

[12]Reginster, J. et al. "Randomized trial of the effects of risedronate on vertebral fractures in women with established postmenopausal osteoporosis." *Osteoporosis International* 2000;11:83-91.

[13]Heaney, R.P. et al. "Risedronate reduces the risk of first vertebral fracture in osteoporotic women." *Osteoporosis International* 2002;13(6):501-5.

[14]McClung, M.R. et al. "Effect of risedronate on the risk of hip fracture in elderly women." Hip Intervention Program Study Group. *New England Journal of Medicine* 2001;344(5):333-340.

[15]Ettinger, B., et al. "Reduction of vertebral fracture risk in postmenopausal women with osteoporosis treated with raloxifene." *Journal of the American Medical Association* 1999;282:637-645.

[16]Neer, R.M. et al. "Effect of parathyroid hormone (1-34) on fractures and bone mineral density in postmenopausal women with osteoporosis." *New England Journal of Medicine.* 2001;344:1434-1441.

[17]Turner, C.H. Review article: "Biomechanics of bone: Determinants of skeletal fragility and bone quality." *Osteoporosis International* 2002; 13 (2):97-104.

[18]Chestnut, C.H. III. et al. "A randomized trial of nasal spray salmon calcitonin in postmenopausal women with established osteoporosis: the prevent recurrence of osteoporotic fractures study." *American Journal of Medicine* 2000;109:267-276.

[19]Lyritis, G.P. et al. "Analgesic effect of salmon calcitonin in osteoporotic vertebral fractures: A double blind placebo controlled clinical study." *Calcified Tissue International* 1991;49:369-372.

[20]Cranney, A. et al. "Calcitonin for preventing and treating corticosteroid-induced osteoporosis." (Cochrane Review). In: *The Cochrane Library*, 2, 2001.

[21]http://courses.washington.edu/bonephys/

[22]Danielson, M.D. et al. "Hip fractures and fluoridation in Utah's elderly population." *Journal of the American Medical Association* 1992;268:746-748.

[23]Jacqmin-Gadda, H. et al. "Fluorine concentrations in drinking water and fracture in the elderly." (letter) *Journal of the American Medical Association* 1995;273:775-6.

[24]Environmental Fact Sheet. Fluoride in Drinking water http://www.des.state.nh.us/factsheets/ws/ws-3-5.htm Landes, L. "America overdosed on fluoride." Available at: http://www.lef.org/fda-museum/8_water/intarticles/fluoride-overdose.html

[25]Hitt, E. "Strontium ranelate decreases incidence of postmenopausal vertebral fractures." *Medscape Medical News* 2002. Available at: http://www.medscape.com/viewarticle/443713

[26]Wuster, C. et al. "Benefits of growth hormone treatment on bone metabolism, bone density and bone strength in growth hormone deficiency and osteoporosis." Department of Internal Medicine Endocrinology and Metabolism, University Medical Clinic Heidelberg, Germany. National Library of Medicine Jan. 15, 2001. http://www.growthhormonetherapy.cc/

[27]Prior, J.C. "Progesterone as a bone-trophic hormone." *Endocrine Reviews* 1990;11:386-398.

[28]Gaby, A. "Progesterone fails Osteoporosis Trial." *Townsend Letter for Doctors and Patients* December 1999. p. 121.

[29]Cundy, T. et al. "Bone density in women receiving depot medroxyprogesterone acetate for contraception." *British Medical Journal* 1991;303:13-16.

[30]Ibid.

[31]Leonetti, H.B. et al. "Transdermal progesterone cream for vasomotor symptoms and postmenopausal bone loss." *Obstetrics and Gynecology* 1999;94:225-228.

[32]Legrain, S. et al. "Dehydroepiandrosterone replacement administration: pharmacokinetic and pharmacodynamic studies in healthy elderly subjects." *Journal of Clinical Endocrinology and Metabolism* 2000;85:3208-17.

[33]Alexandersen, P. et al. "Ipriflavone in the treatment of postmenopausal osteoporosis." *Journal of the American Medical Association* 2000;285(11)1483-8.

CHAPTER 7: The Myth of the Magic Bullet

[1]Van Beresteijn, E.C. et al. "Relation of axial bone mass to habitual calcium intake and to cortical bone loss in healthy early postmenopausal women." *Bone* 1990;11:7-13.

[2]Nordin B.E. "Calcium requirement is a sliding scale." *American Journal of Clinical Nutrition* 2000;71:1381-83.

[3]Hegsted DM. "Calcium and osteoporosis." *Journal of Nutrition* 1986;116:2316-2319.
[4]Ibid.

[5]Anderson, J.B. "The important role of physical activity in skeletal development: how exercise may counter low calcium intake." *American Journal of Clinical Nutrition* 2000;71:1384-6.

[6]Mazess, R.B. "Bone density in premenopausal women: effects of age, dietary intake, physical activity, smoking and birth control pills." *American Journal of Clinical Nutrition* 1991;53:132-42.

[7]Hegsted DM. Ibid.

[8]Mazess, R.B., Ibid.

[9]Dawson-Hughes, B. "Calcium supplementation and bone loss: a review of clinical trials." *American Journal of Clinical Nutrition* 1991; 54:274S-80S.

[10]Patrick. L. "Comparative absorption of calcium sources and calcium citrate malate for the prevention of osteoporosis." http://www.thorne.com/altmedrev/fulltext/calcium4-2.html. (Cited in)

[11]Abelow, B.J. et al.. "Cross-cultural association between dietary animal protein and hip fracture: a hypothesis." *Calcified Tissue International* 1992;50:14-8.

[12]Abelow. B.J et al. Ibid.

[13]Mazess, R.B. et al. "Bone density of the spine and femur in adult white females." *Calcified Tissue International* 1999; 65(2):91-9.

[14]Dibba, B. et al. "Effect of calcium supplementation on bone mineral accretion in Gambian children accustomed to a low-calcium diet." *American Journal of Clinical Nutrition* 2000; 71: 544-9. Aspray T.J. et al, "Low bone mineral content is common but osteoporotic fractures are rare in elderly rural Gambian women." *Journal of Bone and Mineral Research* 1996; 11:1019-25.

[15]Mazees, R. "Bone mineral content of North Alaskan Eskimos." *Journal of Clinical Nutrition* 1974; 27:916-925.

[16]Walker, A. "Osteoporosis and calcium deficiency." *American Journal of Clinical Nutrition* 1965; 16: 327 - 336.

[17]Marsh, A.G., Sanchez, T.V., Mickelsen, O. et al. "Cortical bone density of adult lacto-ovo-vegetarian and omnivorous women." *Journal of the American Dietetic Association* 1980:76:148-151. See also: Ellis, F.R., Holesh, S., Eliss, J.W. "Incidence of osteoporosis in vegetarians and omnivores." *American Journal of Clinical Nutrition* 1972:25:555-58.

[18]NIH Consensus Conference. "Optimal Calcium Intake." NIH Consensus Development Panel on Optimum Calcium Intake. *Journal of the American Medical Association* 1994;272:1942-1944.

Heaney, R. "Distribution of calcium absorption in middle-aged women." *American Journal of Clinical Nutrition* 1986;43:299-305.

[19]Weaver, C., et al. "Dietary calcium: adequacy of a vegetarian diet." *American Journal of Clinical Nutrition* 1994;59(suppl):1238S-41S.

[20]Wyshak,G. "Consumption of carbonated drinks by teenage girls associated with bone fractures." *Archives of Pediatrics and Adolescent Medicine* 2000;154:542-543, 610-613.

[21]Hopper, J.L., Seeman, E. "The bone density of female twins discordant for tobacco use." *New England Journal of Medicine* 1994;330:387-92.

[22]Nordin, B.E. "Calcium requirement is a sliding scale." *American Journal of Clinical Nutrition* 2000;71:1381-83.

[23]Weaver, C.M. Ibid.

[24]Feskanich, D. et al. "Milk, dietary calcium, and bone fractures in women: a 12-year prospective study." *American Journal of Public Health* 1997;87:992-997.

[25]Cumming, R. "Case-Control of risk factors for hip fractures in the elderly." *American Journal of Epidemiology* 1994;139(5):493-503.

[26]Weinsier, R.L. "Dairy foods and bone health: examination of the evidence." *American Journal of Clinical Nutrition* 2000;72:681-9.

[27]Lau, E.M.C. "The epidemiology of hip fracture in Asia: An update." *Osteoporosis International* 1996 Suppl.3:S19-S23.

[28]Kato, I. et al. "Relationship between westernisation of dietary habits and mortality from breast and ovarian cancer in Japan." *Japanese Journal of Cancer Research* 1987; 78:349-57.

[29]Schrezenmeir , J. "Milk and diabetes." *Journal of the American College of Nutrition* 2000; 19(2 Suppl):176S-190S.

[30]Plant, Jane. *Your Life in Your Hands.* Virgin Publishing Ltd, 2000. p.89.

[31]Rusynyk, R.A. "Lactose intolerance." *Journal of the American Osteopathy Association* 2001 Apr;101(4 Suppl Pt I):S10-2.

[32]Plant, Jane. Ibid.

[33]Ibid.

[34]Epstein, S. S. "Unlabeled milk from cows treated with biosynthetic growth hormones: a case of regulatory abdication." *International Journal of Health Services* 1996; 26. (I): 173-85.

CHAPTER 8: Understanding Health

[1]Zhiping, Huang et al. "Nutrition and subsequent hip fracture risk among a national cohort of white women." *American Journal of Epidemiology* 1996;144:124-34.

[2]Cadarette, S.M. et al. "Development and validation of the osteoporosis risk assessment instrument to facilitate selection of women for bone densitometry." *Canadian Medical Association Journal* 2000;162(9):1289-94.

[3]Robinson, E. "Use of hormone replacement therapy to reduce the risk of osteopenia in adolescent girls with anorexia nervosa." *Journal of Adolescent Health* 2000 May;26(5):343.

[4]Mazess, R. et al. "Bone density in premenopausal women: effects of age. Dietary intake, physical activity, smoking and birth control pills." *American Journal of Clinical Nutrition.* 1991;53:132-42.

[5]Baron, J. "Current smoking increases risk of hip fracture in postmenopausal women." *Archives of Internal Medicine* 2001;161:983-988.

[6]National Institutes of Health Osteoporosis and related bone diseases. National Resource Centre. http://www.osteo.org/osteo.html

[7]Tannirandorn, P., Epstein, S. "Drug-induced bone loss." *Osteoporosis International* 2000;11:637-659.

[8]Baudoin, C. et al "Moderate alcohol consumption linked to increased bone mass in elderly women." *American Journal of Epidemiology* 2000;151:773-780.

[9]Cousins, N. *Anatomy of an Illness.* Bantam, 1991.

[10]Gaby, A. *Preventing and Reversing Osteoporosis.* Prima Health 1994.

[11]Eppley, K. et al. *Journal of Clinical Psychology* 1989;45:957-74.

[12]Orme-Johnson, D.W. "Medical care utilization and the Transcendental Meditation Program." *Psychosomatic Medicine* 1987;49:493-507.

[13]Colborn Theo et al. *Our Stolen Future.* Abacus 1997.

[14]Beard, J. et al. "1,1,1-Trichloro-2,2-bis)p-Chlorophenyl)-Ethane (DDT) and reduced bone mineral density." *Archives of Environmental Health* 2000;55(3)177-180.

[15]Glynn, A.W. et al. "Organochlorines and bone mineral density in Swedish men from the general population" *Osteoporosis International* 2000;11:1036-1042.

[16]Cancer Prevention Coalition. Extract from their Consumer Right-to-Know Resolution presented to the UN Food and Ag Org Global Food Summit, Rome. 1998.

CHAPTER 9: Positive Reactions
[1]Cummings, S.R. et al. "Risk factors for hip fracture in white women." *New England Journal of Medicine* 1995;332(12)767-73.

CHAPTER 10: Creating Strong Bones
[1]Calbet, J.A.L. et al. "High bone mineral density in male elite professional volleyball players." *Osteoporosis International* 1999;10:468-474.

[2]Wolff, J.J. et al. "The effect of exercise training programs on bone mass: a meta-analysis of published controlled trials in pre- and postmenopausal women." *Osteoporosis International* 1999;9:1-12.

[3]Bassey, J. "Osteoporosis and Exercise." *Bone Alert* 2000; 6:4-6.

[4]Robertson, M.C. et al. "Effectiveness and economic evaluation of a nurse delivered home exercise programme to prevent falls. A controlled trial in multiple centres." *British Medical Journal* 2001:322:701-704.

[5]Ibid.

[6]Heinonen. A. "High-impact exercise and bones of growing girls: A 9-month controlled trial." *Osteoporosis International* 2000; 11: 1010-1017.

[7]O'Connor, Deirdre. "Osteoporosis." *Alternative Medicine Reviews* 1997;2(1):36. www.thorne.com/altmedrev

[8]TVNZ News Tues., May 8, 2001.

[9]http://www.meltdown.com/osteo2.html

[10]Chopra, Deepak. *Ageless Body, Timeless Mind.* Random House, 1993. p.86.

[11]Fiatarone, M.A. "Exercise training and nutritional supplementation for physical frailty in very elderly people." *The New England Journal of Medicine* 1994;330;25:1769-75.

[12]Gorman, Christine. *Time Magazine* Feb. 5, 2000; 157:5.

[13]CNN; Science Daily. Reported in *Partners, the AIM Magazine* July 1998.

[14]O'Connor, Deirdre. Ibid.

[15]Lumsden, D. B. et al. "Tai chi for osteoarthritis: an introduction for primary care physicians." Geriatrics, 1998;53: 84-88.

[16]Wolf, S.L. et al. "Reducing frailty and falls in older persons: an investigation of Tai Chi and computerized balance training." *Journal of the American Geriatric Society* 1996;44:599-600.

[17]Kerr, et al. "Exercise effects on bone mass in postmenopausal women are site-specific and load dependent." *Journal of Bone and Mineral Research* 1996;11:218-225.

[18]Bennell, K. et al. "The role of physiotherapy in the prevention and treatment of osteoporosis." *Manual Therapy* 2000;5(4):198-213.

[19] Ibid.

[20]New, S. A. "Nutrition and skeletal health. A review of current thinking." Medscape Conference Coverage, based on selected sessions at: The 1st Joint Meeting of the International Bone and Mineral Society and the European Calcified Tissue Society June 5-10, 2001, Madrid, Spain. Available at: http://www.medscape.com/viewprogram/333

[21]Tucker, K.L. et al. "Potassium, Magnesium and fruit and vegetable intakes are associated with greater bone mineral density in elderly men and women." *American Journal of Clinical Nutrition* 1999;64 (4):727-736.

[22]Tucker, K.L. et al. "Bone mineral density and dietary patterns in older adults: The Framingham Osteoporosis Study." *American Journal of Clinical Nutrition* 2002;76(1):245-252.

[23]Sellmeyer, D.E. et al, for the Study of Osteoporotic Fracture. "A high ratio of dietary animal to vegetable protein increases the rate of bone loss and the risk of fracture in postmenopausal women." *American Journal of Clinical Nutrition* 2001;73:118-122.

[24]Remer, T., Manz, F. "Estimation of the renal net acid excretion by adults consuming diets containing variable amounts of protein." *American Journal of Clinical Nutrition* 1994;59:1356-61.

[25]Feskanich D. et al. "Protein consumption and bone fractures in women." *American Journal of Epidemiology* 1996;143:472-79.

[26]Albertazzi, P. et al. "The effect of dietary soy supplementation on hot flushes." *Obstetrics and Gynecology* 1998; 91:6-11.

[27]Gallagher, J.C. et al. Creighton University, Omaha. "The effects of soy isoflavone intake on bone metabolism in post-menopausal women." Presented to symposium on the role of soy in preventing and treating chronic disease. Brussels Belgium, 1996.

[28]Anderson, J.W. et al. "Meta-analysis of the effects of soy protein intake on serum lipids." *New England Journal of Medicine* 1995; 333: 276-82. (A meta-analysis of 38 studies.)

[29]Ingram, D. et al. "Case-control study of phytoestrogens and breast cancer." *Lancet* 1997; 350:990 -94.

[30]Aldercreutz, H. "Phytoestrogens : Epidemiology and a possible role in cancer protection." *Environmental Health Perspectives* 1995; 103(suppl 7):103-112.

[31]Kato, I. et al. "Relationship between westernisation of dietary habits and mortality from breast and ovarian cancer in Japan." *Japanese Journal of Cancer Research* 1987; 78:349-57.

[32]Ho, Suzanne C. Reporting at the Third Annual Scientific Meeting of the Hong Kong Epidemiological Association. Jan 2001.

[33]Horiuchi T. et al. "Effect of soy protein on bone metabolism in postmenopausal japanese women." *Osteoporosis International* 2000;11(8): 721-724.

[34]Nordin, B.E.C. et al. "The nature and significance of the relationship between urinary sodium and urinary calcium in women." *Journal of Nutrition* 1993;123:1615-22.

[35]Harris, S..S. et al. "Caffeine and bone loss in healthy postmenopausal women." *American Journal of Clinical Nutrition* 1994;60:573-8.

[36]Chapuy, M.C. et al. "Vitamin D3 and calcium to prevent hip fractures in elderly women." *New England Journal of Medicine* 1992;327:1637-42.

[37]Buckley, L. M, Hillner, B.E. "Calcium, bisphosphonates cost-effective in preventing fractures in steroid-treated women." *Journal of Rheumatology* 2003;30:132-138.

[38]Trivedi, D.P. et al. "Effect of four monthly oral vitamin D_3 (cholecalciferol) supplementation on fractures and mortality in men and women living in the community: randomised double blind controlled trial." *British Medical Journal* 2003;326:469-472.

[39]Glerup, H. et al. "Commonly recommended daily intake of Vitamin D is not sufficient if sunlight exposure is limited." *Journal of Internal Medicine* 2000:247(2):260-268.

[40]From Medscape News May 8, 2001. Garg, R. et al "Elderly lack adequate levels of Vitamin D." Posted at the American Association of Clinical Endocrinologists 10th Annual Meeting, held in San Antonio, Texas.

[41]Gaby, A. *Preventing and Reversing Osteoporosis.* Prima Health 1994

[42]Sojka, J.E., Weaver, C. "Magnesium Supplementation and Osteoporosis." *Nutrition Reviews* 1995;53(3)71-80.

[43]Geinster, J.Y. et al. "Preliminary report of decreased serum magnesium in postmenopausal osteoporosis." *Magnesium Research* 1989;8:106-9.

[44]Stendig-Lindberg, G. et al. "Trabecular bone density in a two-year controlled trial of peroral magnesium in osteoporosis." *Magnesium Research* 1993;6:155-63.

[45]Dreosti, I.E. "Magnesium status and health." *Nutrition Reviews* 1995;53;7:S23-S27.

[46]Dimai, H.P. et al. "Daily oral magnesium supplementation suppresses bone turnover in young adult males." *Journal of Clinical Endocrinology and Metabolism* 1998; 83 (8): 2742-8.

[47]Jones, G. et al. "Diet in pregnancy linked to bone mineral density in offspring." *European Journal of Clinical Nutrition* 2000;54:749-756.

[48]Heaney, R., Weaver, C. "Calcium absorption from Kale." *American Journal of Clinical Nutrition* 1990;51:656-7.

[49]Healthnotes 2000. www.healthnotes.com

[50]Feskanich, D. et al. "Vitamin K intake and hip fractures in women: a prospective study." *American Journal of Clinical Nutrition* 1999; 69(1):74-9.

[51]Booth, S. et al. "Dietary vitamin K intakes are associated with hip fracture but not with bone mineral density in elderly men and women." *American Journal of Clinical Nutrition* 2000; 71(5):1201-8.

[52]*New Scientist* July 15, 2000. p. 22.

[53]Ibid. 36-7.

[54]Elmstahl, S. et al. "Increased incidence of fractures in middle-aged and elderly men with low intakes of phosphorus and zinc." *Osteoporosis International* 1998;8:333-40.

[55]Eaton-Evans, J. et al. "Copper supplementation and bone mineral density in middle-aged women." Proceedings of the Nutrition Society 1995;54:191A.

[56]Healthnotes 2000. www.healthnotes.com

[57]Neilson, F.H. et al. "Effect of dietary boron on mineral, estrogen and testosterone metabolism in postmenopausal women." *Federation of American Societies for Experimental Biology* (FASEB) 1987;1:394-397.

[58]Newnham, R.E. "The role of boron in human nutrition." *Journal of Applied Nutrition* 1994;46:81-85.

[59]Eisinger, J. et al. "Effects of silicon, fluoride, etidronate, and magnesium on bone mineral density; a retrospective study." *Magnesium Research* 1993;6:247-9.

[60]Healthnotes 2000. www.healthnotes.com

[61]Hyams, D.E. "Scurvy, megalobalstic anaemis and osteoporosis." *British Journal of Clinical Practice* 1963;17:332-340.

[62]Michaëlsson, K. et al. "Serum Retinol Levels and the Risk of Fracture." *New England Journal of Medicine* 2003;348:287-294,347-349.

[63]Melhus, H. "Excessive dietary intake of vitamin A is associated with reduced bone mineral density and an increased risk for hip fracture." *Annals of Internal Medicine* 1998 129(10): 770-8.

[64]Seeman, Ego. "New drugs and new data on old drugs." 22nd Annual meeting of the American Society for bone and mineral research. www.medscape.com

[65]Kruger, M.C. et al. "Calcium, gamma-linolenic acid and iecosapentaenoic acid supplementation in senile osteoporosis." *Aging* 1998;10:385-94.

Index